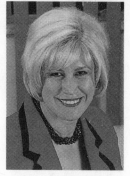

Lily Stojanovska is an Associate Professor in the Faculty of Engineering and Science, Victoria University, Melbourne. For fifteen years Lily has been involved in medical research, developing and teaching under-graduate and post-graduate programs in the areas of health and disease, and supervising post-graduate research students. She is also Director of International Programs for her faculty, responsible for its leadership of overseas programs and promoting collaborations with many overseas universities. She was Director of the University research centre for biotechnology for three and a half years. She has published in scientific journals and has presented her research findings at national and international conferences. She is often an invited speaker on women's health issues at research and educational seminars and a guest speaker at community meetings. She is married and has twin adolescent sons. She has travelled extensively, and lived and worked on three continents. She has a particular love for arts and the theatre. She enjoys reading, walking, cycling and yoga.

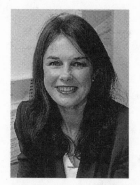

Robyn Craven's particular medical interests are in women's health and epidemiology. She has been involved in the clinical aspects of women's health for over ten years. In her role as Medical Director of the Freemason's Women's Health and Breast Clinic over the last eight years, she has managed the health concerns of women from adolescents to women in their late eighties. She has also been involved in many educational seminars for women and general practitioners. She is a Senior Lecturer in the Department of General Practice at Monash University. She coordinates a Graduate Certificate in Women's Health for post-graduate doctors in Australia and overseas. In addition to being a Fellow of the Royal Australian College of General Practitioners, she has a Masters in Family Medicine and a Graduate Diploma in Clinical Epidemiology. She is currently studying for a Masters Degree in Clinical Epidemiology with a special focus on women's health issues. She is married with four daughters, likes to attend the ballet and opera regularly, loves to read – particularly crime fiction – and tries to keep fit playing tennis and going to the gym.

the other fact of life

taking control of menopause

Robyn Craven and
Lily Stojanovska

A SUE HINES BOOK
ALLEN & UNWIN

First published in 2001

A Sue Hines Book
Allen & Unwin
83 Alexander Street
Crows Nest NSW 2065
Australia
Phone: (61 2) 8425 0100
Fax: (61 2) 9906 2218
Email: info@allenandunwin.com
Web: www.allenandunwin.com

National Library of Australia
Cataloguing-in-Publication entry:

Craven, Robyn.
    The other fact of life: taking control of menopause

    Includes index.

    ISBN 1 86508 550 2.

    1. Menopause. 2. Menopause – Popular works.
    3. Women – Health and hygiene. 4. Women – Australia –

    Interviews. I. Stojanovska, Lily. II. Title.

    612.665

Cover design by Alex Snellgrove
Typeset by Pauline Haas
Printed by Griffin Press, South Australia

10 9 8 7 6 5 4 3 2 1

Contents

Acknowledgements

I wish to thank my friends and family for all their support and interest during the many hours I have spent in writng for the book. In particular my husband Geoff's experienced advice, my daughter Rebecca for her diligent typing of several of the interviews, Tonya and Melanie for spreading the word to their friends and their mothers, and Catherine who is always a delightful support to me.

Thank you, in particular, to our interviewees who have really made the book unique and interesting. My thanks also to our publisher Sue Hines at Allen and Unwin who has developed the concept so well, while maintaining a mature sense of humour. Also, I would like to acknowledge my appreciation of Rachel Lawson, senior editor from Allen and Unwin. She has provided positive and very useful advice and interaction in the final editing of the book.

Robyn Craven

I would like to express my sincere thanks and gratitude to many people that made this book possible. Deep appreciation to all our women interviewees, who enthusiastically agreed to contribute to this book by sharing their personal experiences with us. I thank them for their time, effort, generosity, professionalism and friendship.

I am thankful to our literary agent and editor, Jane Arms, for her editorial expertise, creative thoughts and enthusiasm in the project. I am grateful to Sue Hines, publisher of Allen and Unwin, for embarking on the project before reading a page of it, and Rachel Lawson, senior editor, who played a vital role in making this project possible.

My deep appreciation to Albert McGill for his challenging ideas and helpful comments. I thank my work colleagues at Victoria University for their assistance and support as well as my many friends for their advice and sharing of ideas.

Finally, I would like to thank my family who have supported me and helped me succeed at any venture I have attempted. To my two sons great thanks: to Emil, who has proof read more paragraphs than he cared to read, and to Igor, whose computer knowledge and skills saved me many frustrating hours. To my husband, Alex, for his endless patience, constant source of ideas and gentle guidance. I especially thank him for his love, support and encouragement.

Lily Stojanovska

Introduction

The midlife years are an important stage in women's lives. Many physical and psychological changes take place. For many women it is also a time of reflection, re-evaluation and planning for the future, with more focus and intensity than perhaps ever before. Some have to re-assess their entire way of life in the light of health requirements and general well-being in their older age.

Life expectancy, women's health issues, and the socio-economic status of women in societies such as Australia have changed dramatically over the course of the twentieth century. As little as a hundred years ago the average life expectancy of women was fifty-five. The health of women in the early 1900s was influenced, as it had been for many centuries, by infectious diseases and the complications of childbirth. Now, at the beginning of the twenty-first century, women are living longer than men, with an average life expectancy of over eighty years. Fertility rates have fallen by a third, maternal death rates have halved and female literacy has risen from about half of the male rate to nearly three-quarters of it. Unfortunately, despite their greater longevity, women in most communities continue to report more illness and distress than men.

The World Health Organization's definition of health is: 'a state of complete physical, mental, and social well-being and not merely the absence of disease and infirmity'. The Australian National Women's Health policy, based on recommendations from the World Health Organization, has focused on certain women's issues as being of great importance. These include reproductive health and sexuality, the health of ageing women, emotional and mental health, violence against women, occupational health and safety, the health of women as carers, and the implications for women's health of sex role stereotyping.

Never before have the lives of women at midlife been as complex as they are today. The issues they face are linked with many other factors. While they are contending with the physical changes of midlife and menopause, many women are involved in helping ageing parents or dealing with changes in their relationships with their children and partners or spouses. Many are also involved in part-time or full-time employment. Increasingly, women find that maintaining good health and fitness seems to take more time and effort than when they were younger.

Certain illnesses, such as cancer, particularly breast cancer, osteoporosis, arthritis, hypertension, diabetes, heart disease, and anxiety and depression become more common as women age. The physical changes of ageing, such as weight gain, also affect some women more than others. Fortunately, these physical changes are often compensated for by a more mature and philosophical outlook on life.

One of the principal aims of this book is to encourage women to approach the changes that take place inevitably at midlife in a positive way. In particular, the interviews with women who have dealt with many of the difficulties that most women experience to various degrees at this stage of their lives give insights into the way other women feel and respond to events at their midlife.

The idea for this book was Lily Stojanovska's. She wanted to see how women who had attained visible success in public, business and academic life, and had vigorously continued their careers, had dealt with these midlife challenges. Robyn Craven's interest in the clinical aspects of menopause provided a perfect collaboration. Lily's scientific knowledge, Robyn's clinical experience and their backgrounds in the educational aspects of women's health were the platform for this publication.

We approached each woman by letter, requesting an interview. With the letter we sent a list of questions (see page 249) to set the scene for each conversation. We then met or telephoned the women for a one-on-one interview which took anywhere from forty minutes up to an hour. These were recorded and later transcribed. The interviews in this book reflect conversations that covered twenty, thirty or even forty years of the women's lives and a range of topics. By printing them here as they were transcribed – with all the immediacy and variety of a conversation – it is hoped the reader can experience and interpret similar emotions to those we felt when we conducted the interviews.

The medical chapters give women information on how they can enhance, make informed decisions about, and take more control of their own health. These chapters were based on our clinical and scientific experience with the health concerns of perimenopausal and postmenopausal women.

We both regularly attend international conferences in Australia, Europe, Asia and North America where the latest research in women's health and menopause is presented. That research is conveyed in this book in as honest a way as possible, so that women can decide for themselves what solutions are best for them. We do not set out to convince women of any particular way of thinking or medical regime, but simply to present the state of knowledge as it is today.

These chapters are aimed at women with a certain amount of knowledge – the details here should add to or explain information received from medical and other professionals. A short summary at the beginning of each chapter shows the topics it covers so the reader can choose which chapters are relevant or of interest to them.

The first chapter, 'Hormones', gives an overview of the hormonal changes and symptoms that may occur during the perimenopausal and early postmenopausal years. 'Well-being across cultures' reminds us that responses and experiences are very often culturally determined – it presents epidemiological research that shows that the experience of menopause is quite different in different cultures. Later chapters go beyond the physical symptoms of hot flushes and sweats to examine other experiences such as alteration in libido and psychological symptoms. One of the major concerns of women during their perimenopausal years are the changes they notice in their body shape and weight; the chapters on diet and exercise provide useful guidelines on how to deal with these problems. We go on to cover the longer term consequences of the hormonal changes associated with menopause, such as an increase in the risk of diabetes, heart disease and osteoporosis. Breast cancer is the most common cancer in women, particularly in older age groups, so information on the usual strategies for diagnosis and treatment is included. Finally, the issues surrounding hormone replacement therapy and alternative therapies are discussed in detail.

We hope this up-to-date scientific and medical information will enable women to make responsible choices about the options available to them, to understand how to approach midlife, and to adapt their way of life to eliminate or reduce risks to their minds and bodies. The aim for all women as they enter this phase of their lives should be to improve the quality of their lives and to live these years as happily, actively and productively as they possibly can.

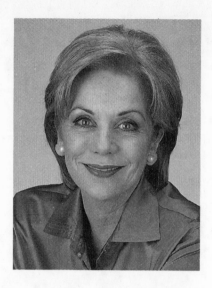

Ita Buttrose, AO, OBE, combines many roles.
She is a businesswoman, journalist, author, media
personality and professional speaker. She is one of
Australia's leading communicators and advises
corporate Australia and community and welfare
organisations. She is Managing Director of Ita
Buttrose Pty Ltd and has published her first
romantic novel. She has also published *A Passionate
Life*, which looks back at her last forty years in the
media and the changes she has seen in Australia, as
well as two other books, *Every Occasion: Your Guide
to Modern Etiquette*, and *Early Edition: My First
Forty Years*. She was made Officer of the Order of
Australia (AO) in 1988 for her services to the
community, particularly in medical education and
health, and received an OBE in 1979 for her services
to journalism. She is patron of many community
and charity organisations and a member of several
professional associations.

Ita Buttrose

I went through menopause at a time when I was busy running my own business and, of course, it was right in the middle of the recession that Australia had to have, so I was really flat out just getting the business to stay profitable. Quite frankly, I was never sure whether my symptoms were related to my work or whether they were related to the menopause. I expect it was a combination of both.

I certainly didn't lack energy. I was working enormously long hours, often from early in the morning until dinner and then late into the night. At that time, it wasn't unusual to get up at five in the morning. If I was tired, I couldn't trace it to the menopause. I would have to say it was work.

But what I did have was the most fearful rage. I definitely had some very strong mood swings – I remember being enormously angry with everybody. Now I tend to accept my problems rather than lay blame elsewhere. After all, life is full of problems. But, back then, I always thought that my anger was connected to nearing menopause.

Then I went to the gynaecologist for my annual check-up and mentioned my anger to him. I could only describe it as an awful rage. He suggested that I take Serapax to help me sleep, but I remembered the terrible effect it once had on my mother and refused his advice.

He got very cross with me and said, 'I suppose you're the sort of woman that wouldn't take hormone replacement therapy if you didn't want to.'

And I said, 'That's right. If I didn't want to, I wouldn't.'

He gave me his rotten prescription, and I threw it out. I'm of the view that my body is mine and, if I don't wish to put anything into it, nobody can make me.

The rage did leave me eventually – maybe my business got less demanding. I wound it up in the end.

Rage is a strong mood though. I'm usually a pretty happy person. I don't suffer from depression, or any of those sorts of things, but I was very depressed at that time. That's why it's very hard for me to decide whether it was my circumstances or the menopause that contributed to my moods. I suspect it was a combination of both.

Did I lose my libido? I find that a most fascinating question. I went to see a menopause specialist, and he gave me a questionnaire. It must have been six or seven pages long. I got to the last page, and it was all to do with sex. Do you have sexual desire? When did you last have sex? How did it feel? Do you ever feel sexy?

I said to him, 'I can't answer this. I'm divorced. I live with my two teenage children and my dog and cat. And I certainly don't walk around having sexual thoughts about them. If there was a bloke around the place I might feel a bit more sexy, but it's a bit hard without one.'

And he said (and I swear it's true), 'What a pity that so many women like you live alone when there are so many available men in Australia.'

I certainly have sexual thoughts. I just wrote a chapter for a book I'm working on at the moment, and I got so horny I had to stop writing.

As a journalist, I've grown up discussing all sorts of issues around menopause. We used to run menopause seminars and write often about the menopause. There's no magazine around that discusses the issue to the depths that we used to. After all, I've talked to Australians about their sexual habits (when I chaired the National Advisory Committee on AIDS), so I don't have a problem discussing these things with people. I don't believe they are taboo subjects.

The menopause is something all women experience and unless we can talk about it openly we will never be able to get women to realise it's not something we need to suffer in silence. It's a fact of life and a very important one. I think it's also very liberating. I haven't met a woman anywhere who has mentioned her 'empty womb' when discussing menopause. I think that we are all absolutely delighted that we won't be having any more children.

While I've often discussed the subject of menopause in my public life, I didn't speak about it much from a personal level while I was going through it. I probably had so many other problems to juggle that I just kept battling on and struggling to overcome all the things that were overwhelming me.

After the Serapax incident, I decided that doctors were generally hopeless and I'd just manage on my own. And that's what I did. I made sure I had a regular massage and tried to walk every morning. That was about as much as I could manage at the time because my work commitments were enormous.

Like a lot of small business operators, I was clearly overworked, and I had far too much on my plate. I was doing so many jobs just trying to keep the company going. I was pretty exhausted at the end of it, like so many other Australian business people at the time who were experiencing the same pressures.

I also suffered from insomnia. This could have been because of my rotten job, but I had read that your sleep patterns become disturbed during menopause.

In the end I decided that the cause didn't really matter all that much. What really mattered was the way I handled the situation. I'd be lying there in the middle of the night and I'd think, Oh, damn, I'm awake. I'll just keep lying here. Then I'd remind myself of stories I'd read about how you need less sleep as you get older, and I'd try to think positively about the insomnia.

Other symptoms of the menopause didn't bother me at all. I got a couple of hot flushes, and they were a bit nerve-wracking. Everyone else was saying how cold it was, and I was thinking, Oh, God, it's one of these dreaded hot flushes. But I only got a few of them, so they were nothing much. I just sat there very still and took my coat off.

Growing old is a pain in the butt. We all have to pretend we don't mind, but what a lie that is. Unless you go to a plastic surgeon and have a nip and tuck, or whatever they all get done, what else can you do about it?

I think it's important to keep fit. I try to keep my weight under control, and I do a lot of walking. I'm careful with what I eat, and I think my health is pretty good. Actually, it's excellent.

You have to think positive. I find it riveting when my hairdresser tells me that people are convinced I've had a face-lift. I haven't had one bit of cosmetic surgery. I come from good genetic stock, and I'm very happy in my life. I think that's what makes you look good.

I worry about all these women who rush off and have plastic surgery. Who are they fooling? You see them sometimes, these poor old ladies, who have had so many face-lifts. Their faces might look young, but they walk like old women. I don't have a problem with women who opt for plastic surgery. If that's what they want to do, then they should do it – it's their choice, and I think that's important. But it's not my choice.

I'm a well-built woman, I know, but I definitely needed to lose some excess weight last year. I decided that I just wasn't happy being overweight anymore – that extra stone was just too much. I think at menopause you really have to be serious about a low-fat diet. I combine this with a daily walk for up to an hour if I can manage it. While I still allow myself to have a couple of glasses of wine, these days I'm much more conscious of what I put in my mouth.

Obesity is such an enormous health problem in Australia, and it's a major cause of arthritis, hip replacements, those sorts of things. I want to enjoy my old age, and the only way to do that is to remain fit.

I wasn't greatly troubled by my periods, but it's nice not to bother about them anymore. It's great to be free. I read about these women around sixty having babies. Imagine getting up for the two-year-old's bottle at sixty-two.

These days I feel very optimistic and confident that there's still nothing I can't do. I have goals that I want to achieve, and I intend to reach them all. It helps when you've acquired a bit of wisdom along the way.

As you become older, you certainly re-evaluate your financial status. Now we are all living longer, and it's clear that governments are not going to be able to provide Australians with pensions in the way they once did.

Women's financial independence is even more crucial, because we continue to out-live men. I think now is a time to decide how much longer you need to work and how much more you need to save. I am kept busy as a writer and TV personality and enjoy the freedom to choose when, and how, I will retire.

I think my friends have become a very important part of my life now. They were always important, of course, but I've really begun to appreciate the value of my friendships, especially my female friends. I've found my women friends are very solid and supportive, and I love their company.

Five of us, all in our fifties, went on a farm holiday for a couple of weeks last year. We had the most fantastic time. We went out and toured all day, then sat around the big fire in the evening and talked about all sorts of things over some wine and food.

Once you're over fifty-five, you do start thinking about the pleasures of retirement. But these days, many women and men of my generation, including myself, have children who are still living at home, and elderly parents to care for.

My father is eighty-nine, and I manage his household and organise every aspect of his life. With my son at home, it can become very demanding, especially when you are still working as well. It's also difficult because Dad has some dementia, and he can't see or hear very well. It's a big responsibility, and he doesn't want to go into a home. It's probably too late now, but Dad should have thought about all of this when he was seventy.

Growing older is something we all have to face eventually, and it's bound to be a new challenge. I think governments have a very poor track record on acknowledging the enormous impact the aged population is going to have on all of us. We all have to take responsibility for our older age – there's just no question about it.

Over the next few decades, I hope I'm going to become disgustingly rich. Now I haven't got children to put through school any more, I'm free. I've done all the things I've always wanted to do. I've always supported the children, put them through school and university, and now I only have to worry about me. I hope to become more successful as an author. I've had four books published, and now I'm writing my fifth, a novel.

I've tried hormone replacement therapy. I absolutely hated it. While I took it, I felt nauseated and suffered headaches, so I gave it all up. Now I take a plant hormone called Remifemin, which has just been approved by the Therapeutic Good Association as a treatment for menopause.

My grandmother lived until she was ninety-six, my mother until eighty, and all my aunts and uncles are alive and kicking. So it looks like my options for a long life must be pretty good. And there's plenty to do to fill the years.

Chapter One
Hormones

When does menopause begin? Symptoms you might experience during menopause. The hormones in your body, including oestrogen and progesterone, and how they work. How changing hormones might affect you. Some general strategies for coping successfully with menopause.

Menopause defines the end of a woman's reproductive life. Most women cope very well with this stage of their lives, but some women regret the loss of their ability to have children. Others are happy to leave behind worries about contraception and the discomforts of the monthly menstrual cycle.

The usual age range for the onset of menopause is from forty-five to fifty-five, with the average age of onset at around fifty. The biological function of the ovaries has changed very little over the centuries and despite improvements in the life expectancy of women, particularly during the twentieth century, this average age of onset has remained constant.

Menopause occurring any time between forty and sixty years, however, is still within the normal range, but women who experience menopause in their early forties are often thought to be too young for it, and women in their late fifties without menopausal symptoms worry that they are abnormal.

Menopause before the age of forty is regarded as premature and occurs naturally at that time in a small number of women. In rare cases, young women in their late teens, twenties or early thirties may experience premature menopause. Genetic or hereditary factors play a role in determining when menopause occurs, and family history is often a predictor of early menopause. Some women in this group stop having regular menstrual cycles for other reasons, such as significant weight loss, stress, excessive exercise, medications that affect ovarian function, or illnesses. Once these have been sorted out, menstruation usually starts again spontaneously.

Smoking affects the age of onset of menopause. Just as it adversely affects the lungs and blood vessels, chronic smoking has a toxic effect on the ovaries and lowers oestrogen levels throughout a woman's reproductive life. Other factors influencing the age of onset of menopause include living at high altitudes and, possibly, having a vegetarian diet.

Women who have had a large number of children may have menopause later than other women, but this association is not completely conclusive.

The premenopausal phase in a woman's normal reproductive life is when periods are regular and no menopausal symptoms are present. In most women this is from mid-teens to early forties. The perimenopause is the time prior to menopause (it may last four to five years or more), when periods become irregular and symptoms of menopause, such as hot flushes, start to occur.

Most women would like to predict the start of menopause, particularly if they are experiencing poor health during the perimenopausal years – those occurring immediately before menopause sets in. Unfortunately, measuring hormone levels can only provide a guide to what is happening within the ovary, because there are marked fluctuations in a woman's hormone levels in the years leading up to menopause. There is no specific test to determine when a woman's last period will occur.

In the four or five years on average leading up to their last menstrual period, many women start to notice some physical and psychological changes. These symptoms can include hot flushes and night sweats, palpitations, fatigue, irritability and mild depressive symptoms. These changes are usually caused by fluctuations in the production of hormones from the ovaries.

The cessation of periods is called 'amenorrhoea'. Menopause is said to have occurred after one year of amenorrhoea, but, occasionally, ovulation will occur even after twelve months of amenorrhoea and can cause a recurrence in menstrual bleeding. Most women will usually notice some premenstrual symptoms before bleeding starts again. This is the result of a temporary resurgence in their ovarian hormones. Breast discomfort, bloating and pain in the lower abdomen are common symptoms of this. If postmenopausal bleeding occurs one year or more after the last period, you should see your doctor, as it is important to exclude cancer of the uterus as a cause of the bleeding.

'All my life I've been doing things that I think I'm quite good at. Now I'm trying to tackle activities that are more challenging.'

JAN WADE

Some women may continue to produce oestrogen from the ovary, even though ovulation has ended. This hormone production may last for one or two years after menopause. Weaker oestrogens may also be produced from other areas in the body, such as from fatty tissue. (For example, a hormone from the adrenal gland is changed into a weak oestrogen, called oestrone, in fatty tissue.) Women who are overweight may continue to produce higher levels of oestrogen than thinner women, which has advantages and disadvantages. In women who produce oestrone there may be less bone loss and possibly protection against the brain changes that lead to the development of Alzheimer's Disease. These are discussed further in the chapters on Alzheimer's disease and osteoporosis.

Surgical menopause is the removal of the ovaries through an operation, usually because of disease in or around the ovaries.

Endometriosis, ovarian cysts, or more rarely cancer of the ovary or uterus, are reasons for the ovaries to be removed.

Surgical removal of the ovaries precipitates young women into menopause, and these women will suffer serious adverse symptoms that can affect their quality of life if oestrogen replacement therapy is not, or cannot, be given.

Women who experience a natural menopause have time to adjust to the changes in their bodies as they move through their perimenopausal years. In contrast, women who become menopausal through surgery have very little time to adjust mentally or physically to the sudden loss of their ovarian function and the symptoms this produces. These women are likely to experience sudden severe hot flushes and night sweats. Women in this situation should discuss options for hormone replacement with their doctor. Young women usually require quite different hormone replacement treatment – and doses – from older women who have had a naturally occurring menopause.

'Consistently hot flushes I could almost tolerate. What I could not abide were my general mood swings and feeling crabby and not being on top of things.'

STEPHANIE ALEXANDER

There are a variety of symptoms commonly experienced in the perimenopausal years – those leading up to menopause. Some of these are directly related to the ovarian hormonal changes. The hot flushes and night sweats result from either a fall in oestrogen levels or persistently low oestrogen levels. The exact role that oestrogen plays in the production of hot flushes and sweats is not clearly known, but oestrogen is known to interact with other substances within the brain, resulting in the brain's temperature control becoming unstable. For most women, oestrogen replacement therapy helps control these symptoms.

Other symptoms may be more related to the sleep disturbance caused by hot flushes, night sweats or fluctuating hormones. Many women complain of fatigue, irritability and mild depression. Some-times these symptoms are severe, seriously affecting women's quality of life and well-being. But each person's perimenopause and menopause is unique and what your friends or relatives experience may be very different from what you experience.

Most women cope very well with their symptoms. Even those with significant changes in their hormones somehow manage to continue their daily lives. Some of the women we interviewed reported few noticeable symptoms and others had unique experiences. Despite their varied responses, all our interviewees managed to fulfil their commitments, simply learning ways to cope and adjust along the way.

Throughout the child-bearing years, from early adolescence to menopause, two hormones in the pituitary gland, follicle stimulating hormone (FSH) and luteinising hormone (LH), stimulate the ovaries. During each menstrual cycle, these hormones promote the production of one or more eggs in the ovary. These developing eggs produce oestrogen.

Oestrogen levels reach a peak about mid-cycle, usually around day fourteen in a twenty-eight-day cycle. Ovulation generally occurs about this time. Some women who are in tune with their bodies are aware of their ovulation times when oestrogen thickens the endometrium or the lining of the uterus. Around ovulation there are also changes in the tissue lining the vagina and cervix and changes in mucus production in the vagina. Some women notice that their normal vaginal secretions become more like an egg white consistency around this time and associate these changes in mucus with the fertile stage of their cycle. Changes in mucus secretion can be used to plan or avoid pregnancy.

In the last fourteen days of the menstrual cycle, the ovary produces another hormone called progesterone. It generally reaches a peak around day twenty-one of a normal twenty-eight-day cycle. Women who are trying to become pregnant can take a blood sample to measure the level of progesterone in the blood at this time to help determine whether ovulation has occurred.

Progesterone also acts on the endometrial lining of the uterus, changing it from a state called 'proliferative' endometrium, where the lining is continually thickening either in preparation for implantation of a fertilised egg or, in the very late stage of a non-pregnant cycle, to a state of 'secretory' endometrium, which leads to menstrual bleeding. If the egg is not fertilised, the ovary produces decreasing levels of oestrogen and progesterone, which results in the shedding of the endometrial lining of the uterus and a normal menstrual period.

From their early to mid forties, many women start to notice that their menstrual cycles become closer together, sometimes only two to three weeks apart. This may concern some women, particularly if the short cycles are associated with heavy bleeding. As discussed earlier, the phase in women's reproductive lives when cycles start to significantly change and symptoms start to occur is called perimenopause and this generally lasts from four to five years.

'I guess menopause just slid by me in many ways because the changes coincided with so many other turbulent changes taking place in my life such as remarriage, new career directions and the busy and complex demands of family life with adult children.'

ELAINE CANTY

It is not uncommon for women who have these frequent heavy periods to become low in their stores of body iron, or even to develop anaemia as a result of iron deficiency. Frequent, heavy periods can be debilitating, especially if anaemia occurs, and excessive tiredness as well as the frustration associated with frequent periods are common complaints.

Women who are suffering as a result of frequent periods or heavy bleeding should consult their doctor. There are a number of good treatments available to help with problem or heavy bleeding. It is also important to know whether the symptoms that you are experiencing are normal or abnormal. Some women who continue to have severe problems with their periods in their forties or early fifties may need to have a hysterectomy. But in many situations medication is all that is needed.

Hysterectomy solves the problems of heavy bleeding and pain related to menstruation during the perimenopausal years, but many women do not understand that some of their other symptoms, such as hot flushes and sweats, will not change if their uterus is removed but the ovaries are left. Hysterectomy only stops the symptoms directly caused by menstrual bleeding.

Menopausal symptoms such as hot flushes and sweats are the result of changes in ovarian hormones, particularly oestrogen. The function of the ovaries, particular in the regular development of egg follicles significantly declines during perimenopause and oestrogen levels may fluctuate considerably during this time.

Essentially, menopause occurs because there are few or no eggs left in the ovaries, and they become unresponsive to stimulation by the pituitary gland hormones FSH and LH. At the start of reproductive life in early adolescence, the ovaries start off with several hundred thousand egg follicles. Most of these eggs die off spontaneously and never undergo full maturation to ovulation. Only about four to five hundred eggs ever develop to the point of ovulation throughout the child-bearing years.

By the time most women reach their early forties, only a few thousand eggs are left in the ovary. These ageing follicles tend to decrease at a much faster rate than previously.

A woman's ability to become pregnant is much lower by the age of forty. Even if eggs are being regularly produced, it is more difficult for these ageing eggs to become fertilized, and pregnancy rates are much lower in women at this age. Women in their twenties or thirties with regular menstrual cycles find that it is much easier to become pregnant, compared with women with regular cycles in their late thirties and forties. It is important for women who are delaying pregnancy until they are older to be aware that this may affect their ability to conceive.

However, even if there is only one egg left in the ovary, there is potentially a risk of pregnancy occurring and it is important to continue with contraception for twelve months after the last period.

In the late perimenopause very long menstrual cycles, from three to eleven months apart, may occur. Oestrogen, FSH and other hormone levels fluctuate considerably during perimenopause, and this is the reason behind many of the symptoms, both physical and psychological, that women experience.

When oestrogen levels are persistently low, hot flushes and night sweats may occur. Once these symptoms disappear, congested, painful swollen breasts and abdominal bloating often replace them. It is also common for a prolonged heavy menstrual bleed, often lasting two to three weeks, to follow a period of amenorrhoea.

Commonly, the normal cyclical hormonal balance between oestrogen and progesterone is disturbed. An excessive level of oestrogen, which contributes to the thickening of the endometrial lining, may build up if it is not balanced by an equal level of progesterone production in the later stages of the menstrual cycle.

In some of these erratic cycles, ovulation only occurs after two to three months of unopposed oestrogen production or it may not occur at all. This results in a very heavy menstrual loss from an endometrial lining that has not been exposed to an adequate dose of progesterone. Many women will need to take progestogens (a synthetic form of progesterone) to correct this temporary hormonal imbalance.

The level of FSH tends to increase in the years leading to menopause. Even in women with regular cycles and normal levels of oestrogen throughout the cycle, FSH levels for premenopausal women are above normal.

The ovary produces a number of hormones and other hormone-like substances, one of which is inhibin. When the ovary produces high levels of oestrogen and inhibin, the production of FSH from the pituitary gland is inhibited to some degree. Inhibin levels tend to decline in the perimenopausal phase, which is one of the reasons why FSH levels start to rise, despite regular cycles.

Typically, however, the levels fluctuate too much to rely on measuring these hormones in perimenopausal or postmenopausal women. The decision to use hormone replacement therapy to allay symptoms of menopause centres around whether or not symptoms are bothersome. A low oestrogen level on its own is not a sufficient reason to prescribe oestrogen replacement therapy.

The ovary also produces the male hormone testosterone, but it is produced at much lower levels than in men. Testosterone is an important hormone for libido. In excess amounts, it can be associated with excessive hair growth on the face and body (hirsutism) and acne, although some women with acne and hirsutism have an increased sensitivity to normal levels of testosterone within the hair follicles and sebaceous glands.

'There are some differences in my life from ten years ago, but I don't think that this is due to menopause, but simply growing older and hopefully gaining some wisdom along the way.'

BARBARA CHAMPION

Testosterone production and blood levels decline gradually in women as they age, as they do in men. Women who have their ovaries removed early may need testosterone and oestrogen replacement therapy to maintain their sex drive and general well-being.

In women who experience a natural menopause, the post-menopausal ovary predominately produces more testosterone than oestrogen, although levels are lower than in premenopausal women. The benefits of adding testosterone to oestrogen replacement has still not been clearly defined by adequately controlled clinical studies. The problem is that sexuality, sexual desire and libido are complex and do not necessarily correlate with hormone levels. Linking a decline in sexual function to hormone-related causes inevitably means that some women may be inappropriately treated with hormones when other factors, such as marital conflict or depression, may be responsible.

The symptoms most clearly attributable to menopause are hot flushes and vaginal dryness, but other symptoms may also be present. Some women may be concerned about palpitations, which can occur with or without hot flushes, but these symptoms may not be automatically attributable to menopause. Some women experience dry, irritable skin or a feeling like ants crawling on the skin called formication.

Changes in oestrogen levels can have widespread effects on the body and can affect nerve function, resulting in short-term memory disturbances. Many women who are concerned by problems with memory find that hormone replacement therapy is beneficial. Of course, if frequent night sweats and hot flushes are interrupting your sleeping patterns, leaving you tired and irritable, this can also affect your memory and concentration.

'By the time I had moved into the role of Premier, the symptoms had become a little more manageable, but I did often wonder how Jeff Kennett would have coped with the same circumstances.'

JOAN KIRNER

Short-term memory loss at menopause does not signal the onset of Alzheimer's disease. It is usually a temporary disturbance resulting from a lack of sleep and a minor disturbance in the function of the nerve cells in the brain that are associated with memory. There is a possible relationship between Alzheimer's disease and low oestrogen levels in women later in life, and we discuss this further in our chapter on Alzheimer's disease.

There are many misconceptions about menopause, including a belief that all women suffer at menopause, that all women have negative attitudes to menopause and that most women seek medical advice for menopausal problems.

Although a number of women experience hot flushes and other symptoms around menopause, they do not bother most women. Perhaps 10 to 20 per cent will experience severe debilitating hot flushes and will need to seek help and treatment for them.

Some women regret the end of their reproductive lives. Others, particularly if they have experienced significant discomfort with menstruation, are very pleased to see an end to their monthly periods.

Poor general or psychological health may exacerbate menopausal symptoms and make it more difficult for women to cope. Women may also experience many stresses in their lives at this time, such as difficult (or even normal) adolescent children, ageing parents, marital conflict, and financial or employment hardship, and these may affect their general health.

Feeling that you have control over your life, even if this is not the reality, is important. Personality plays an important role in maintaining control in difficult situations, and hardy people, or people who have developed useful coping strategies, are less likely to become ill or suffer from adverse symptoms of menopause.

Everyone can learn to cope. If you feel you are not coping or your stress levels are adversely affecting your health, support and advice from a counsellor or psychologist may be helpful.

People who feel powerless or lack control over their lives are more prone to illnesses such as chronic depression. Women who are involved in active part-time or full-time employment outside their roles as mothers, wives or daughters often have more confidence and self-esteem. Interacting with other women of a similar age who are experiencing similar challenges is helpful.

At this time of life we are all faced with friends and relatives of a similar age to ours who develop serious, life-threatening illnesses. We often forget that, at the beginning of the last century, the life expectancy of women was fifty-five, and women were dying as a result of complications at childbirth and from infectious diseases. Improvements in public health and antenatal care have had a significant effect on the death rate. Today, cancers and heart disease are the more common causes of illness and death and, although women's life expectancy is now around eighty years of age, not everyone is lucky enough to live this long.

Menopause signals a time to re-evaluate the way you live. Stopping smoking, correcting a poor diet and aiming for daily regular exercise are important. Changes in body shape and an increase in weight, particularly around the abdomen, occur commonly in women from forty onwards. Genetics probably plays a role in weight changes as well and, occasionally, hormones such as an underactive thyroid gland are responsible.

Despite other contributing factors, most of us tend to eat more and exercise less. Many women blame weight gain during these years on hormone replacement therapy, but this is often not the case. Several studies have shown that women on hormone therapy actually gain less weight than those not on it. The PEPI (Postmenopausal Estrogen/Progestin Intervention) study, conducted over three years in the US, compared the changes in women on hormone replacement therapy with those in women not taking it. The results showed that there was an overall weight gain in both groups of women. Women on hormone replacement therapy, however, gained about a kilogram less than women who were not using it.

At menopause, it is important to maintain regular pap smears to screen for cervical cancer and regular mammograms for breast cancer detection.

Although most women have positive attitudes towards menopause, they are often concerned about menopause as a sign of old age. A positive attitude towards ageing is important, and many women at this stage of life who find themselves free of child-rearing responsibilities develop or extend their careers. This period of women's lives can be a time of great productivity.

Exciting career options can be developed, many women return to further education and others use their new-found financial freedom as an opportunity for travel.

There is a myth that women develop depression in response to what is called the 'empty-nest syndrome', when their children leave home to study or work. Women are often happier and have better marital relationships and harmony after their children have left home.

Many of the symptoms experienced by women at menopause are short-lived. Only a small proportion of women have hot flushes and sweats that persist for any length of time, and most women find that hot flushes and sweats become less frequent over time. Hormone replacement therapy is very effective for moderate to severe hot flushes and sweats. Many women try either alternative therapies or supplements for milder symptoms. Women who have commenced hormone therapy for symptoms can stop their therapy at any time if they wish.

Vaginal dryness, which may cause discomfort with sexual intercourse, is a characteristic of lower oestrogen levels in older women. This can be readily treated with an oestrogen therapy used specifically in the vagina and does not necessarily need additional oral or skin-patch oestrogen treatments.

Some women seem more predisposed to psychological symptoms, such as mild depression, fatigue, lack of concentration and irritability, than others. These symptoms may be the result of a life-time sensitivity to hormonal changes and often become evident at those times in our lives when hormones are changing more rapidly, such as the postnatal depression experienced after childbirth. Hormone replacement therapy may be helpful for women who are prone to psychological symptoms. Other treatments may also be needed, and these are discussed further in the chapter on hormones, psychology and the female reproductive cycle.

Postmenopausal women may be at risk of developing osteoporosis, higher cholesterol levels and have a decreased ability to metabolise carbohydrates and sugar, making them prone to premature heart disease and diabetes. These issues will be discussed in subsequent chapters.

Most women are not likely to experience unpleasant symptoms during the perimenopausal years. If you do have problems, whether minor or severe, seek advice from friends, family members, colleagues, doctors or other health professionals.

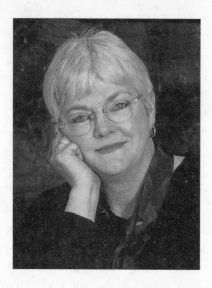

For twenty-one years, before it closed on New Year's Eve 1997, 'Stephanie's Restaurant' was acclaimed as one of the best in the country and an essential Melbourne experience for visitors and residents alike. A regular contributor to *The Age* and *Australian Table*, Stephanie Alexander, OAM, has written many books, among them *Stephanie's Australia, Stephanie's Seasons, Recipes My Mother Gave Me* and the classic *The Cook's Companion*. In 1998, in collaboration with Maggie Beer, she published *Stephanie Alexander and Maggie Beer's Tuscan Cookbook* and in the following year wrote, presented and produced the seven-part series on Australian food and wine for ABC television entitled *A Shared Table*. Through her writing, teaching and public advocacy, Stephanie Alexander has remained a champion of Australian produce and of the importance in our day-to-day lives of good food. Stephanie is also a consultant and partner at the Richmond Hill Cafe and Larder in Melbourne.

Stephanie Alexander

I missed a period quite early. I was about forty-four, or forty-five. I know exactly when it was because I was travelling in Europe, and I went to see my gynaecologist before I left, because I had missed a period and I had been getting headaches. She just asked me to keep a little diary of what was happening to me, and as I was going away for four weeks I had some time to think about myself and to actually note the symptoms.

So I did that, and it was in that time away that I started to experience really serious flushes, which were amazingly continuous, and for the first time I started to get a really extraordinary hangover if I drank too much wine, which would turn into a sort of migraine. This has become a continuing symptom for me. I would get the deserved seediness after a big night and a headache that just didn't go away. It didn't respond to any Aspirin, or anything, and that was a surprise. I didn't know what had hit me, because I had never had headaches like these before.

When I came back and went and saw my gynaecologist, she said it is really quite common, so that was the start of it. I don't think I had any psychological thing about menopause one way or the other.

I went on to hormone replacement therapy because the hot flushes were very consistent and I was working very hard. I didn't have drenching sweats, or anything, but I really didn't sleep very well and I was constantly disturbed – getting up and wandering around the house a couple of times during the night and just not feeling great.

What has amazed me is that I've had two goes at going off hormone replacement therapy in about fourteen years and both times I felt so frightful that I went back on it. The last time was December 2000. I thought, I can't possibly be still having these symptoms, because they've been going on for so long. My gynaecologist reduced the dose at one point, and the symptoms did not reappear, but every now and again I think I've been on it for too long. You talk to people who say it's really bad to take it for any length of time.

I had one go without hormone replacement therapy that lasted for about one month, and my doctor was quite supportive of that, but eating soy products and taking evening primrose oil did nothing, so I went back on it. And then, as I said, I tried again in 2000.

I go to a gym and the gym instructor was particularly influenced by the reports that say it's bad for you to be on hormone replacement therapy, and it got to me eventually. So I thought, How do I know I'm still having these symptoms? So I went off it again, and within five or six days I had all the symptoms again. It was bizarre. Consistently hot flushes I could almost tolerate. What I could not abide were my general mood swings and feeling crabby and not being on top of things. So I went back on it again.

I discussed what was going on with my friends, rather than my family, although I probably spoke a bit to my sister who had had a hysterectomy when she was relatively young, and she thought that she didn't have any symptoms. But I certainly talked about it with friends my own age – we all went to university together – and I was certainly well ahead of them in terms of symptoms. But now they've all gone through it.

One is on hormone replacement therapy. One just struggled through without saying much at all – maybe she didn't find it all too terrible. Another found it an easy transition. She really didn't have any symptoms, although she had some thinning of the hair, but she said she didn't feel different emotionally. I didn't talk to my kids about it because it didn't seem to be very relevant, but it wasn't a taboo topic.

I still managed to do what I had to do, but menopause made me feel a bit ratty. When I was on hormone replacement therapy I felt more energetic. The main symptoms were the hot flushes and the frightful headaches, which were triggered by drinking red wine, and which I still get occasionally despite being on hormone replacement therapy.

The headaches are really disturbing. I thought I had a brain tumour, which I haven't. I'm not talking about drinking two bottles of wine a day, but maybe two-thirds of a bottle once every few weeks. These terrible headaches can last for two or three days, and they don't respond to anything. I find that very hard.

When I went to see a physician about what I thought was a brain tumour, he asked me, of course, if I was on hormone replacement therapy, and I said I had been but was not at the moment – the consultation must have coincided with one of my moments when I was about to go off it – and he said you may find you may never have another headache.

I don't think that's happened, because when I went off it at Christmas time I only lasted for three weeks. I just felt generally not able to cope. I later repeated the experiment over a month period. Again I started to feel very weepy, slept badly and had frequent hot flushes. So I went back on it.

As far as other symptoms go, I did suffer from a bit of lack of concentration, and I also lack confidence judging distance. I don't enjoy driving very much any more, not that I was ever a petrol head, but these days I go out of my way to take taxis rather than drive. It's a lack of confidence, and I do think I don't judge distances correctly any more.

I don't think I ever thought very much about the effect menopause would have on me in the beginning. I did think about growing old, and I do feel reasonably content. I say to myself, Well, I'm nearly sixty, and I cannot go on forever, and I do feel relatively comfortable. The menopause is just a different part of being alive. But I do have a vague anxiety about how I am going to cope when I'm eighty-four and until

I become very old. My father's ninety, so I'm in the middle of coping with my own parent. I think it's very sad losing your capability and independence and not being completely on the ball mentally and knowing you are just not able to do things that you once did. Women seem to cope with it better than men.

I'd say I have recently been through ten really tough years, and I do feel a sense of release at having dealt with them. I got through them. I achieved what I had to achieve. I can relax now feeling that I am in control of my own destiny, and that's quite nice. It intrigues me that it can take so long to get to that position in life.

Apart from these shocking headaches, my energy levels are as high as they have ever been. I go to the gym regularly, but there are some physical signs – every now and then I realise it is hard to get up from this or that position, and it gives me a shock. But I don't believe that I have lost energy or drive. I am enjoying my life so much more now because I no longer have financial and emotional stresses.

Most people think they have done their most important work in their fifties, but I don't think I have. I feel quite positive. My friends and I talk about it and maybe I can solve the old age problem creatively too.

I have a fantasy – and I have a history of making my fantasies work – that there is a community of intelligent people out there who could somehow live together communally as older people, so that they can provide company and stimulation for each other. It's a huge problem, as we know, but somehow I'm going to try and make a stab at dealing creatively with the last part of my life.

I have put on a lot of weight in my menopause. Recently I had my cholesterol done, and it was a bit too high (5.9), and I was told to go on a low-fat diet. I believe I eat very healthily, but it's not what a doctor would call a strictly low-fat diet. I eat well, I exercise regularly and I don't eat junk food, but I consistently put on a couple of kilos a year. That's very depressing.

Since the time when I first noticed symptoms of menopause when I was travelling in Europe I would say I'm now 8–9 kilos heavier, and that's ten years later, and yet I feel very healthy. I rarely get a cold, I don't get any of the viruses that other people get, I don't get stomach upsets, but I get itches – everybody gets something – and I know I've got a very strong constitution. I just can't control my weight.

I may be a lot heavier than I was when I was thirty, but I would say I'm emotionally much better than I was then, and I live a much healthier life. Once upon a time, I would sit around drinking with staff once or twice a week until two or three in the morning. Now I'm in bed by ten or eleven.

I pushed myself at thirty. I was burning candles at every possible end: I had a bad marriage, I was running a restaurant at its most difficult time, and working stupid hours because there didn't seem to be any alternative. I would say I'm much happier and much saner now than when I was thirty.

As far as exercise goes, I used to be the absolute couch potato. It was only four years ago that I found a little gym that was very near where I lived, and I could walk there. I have continued to go and found that gradually I have got to really enjoy it. Now I go three times a week.

Around the start of my menopause, I was quite unhappy. I was very short tempered because of the hours I was working and the situation I was in. It was a tense time, but I don't believe it had much to do with my hormonal state.

My circumstances certainly made me feel unhappy a lot of the time, and I did probably burden my close friends with my emotional worries. It was also a time of financial difficulties, and I had emotionalised these financial worries. All in all, it was a pretty nasty combination, but I did have a lot of support from my friends.

I think the choice to take hormone replacement therapy is a very personal matter. Some people do, and others, like a very dear friend of mine who's into biodynamic agriculture, are appalled by the idea. This friend lent me a very persuasive book on the subject, which I read. I think that's probably why I went off it at an earlier time. In the end, of course it's horses for courses. If you're one of those people that have one hot flush in fifteen years, you don't need it.

My bones are excellent (having had a bone density test), so for me it's just dealing with the headaches. I'd like to feel that the next ten years could be really creative and positive; I'll definitely write more. I'm trying to come to terms with the fact that I don't need to work as hard, either financially, or for any other reasons. If I don't have any appointments before 10.30, I can go to the gym, read the paper, something like that. I'd like to feel I can build into the next twenty or thirty years the space and the time so, if I wanted to, I could go and learn a language. I like travelling with a good travelling companion.

The next ten years look really positive. I don't know what will happen after that. As I said before, my father is ninety and his father died at ninety-six, so I've got good genes.

Chapter Two
Well-being across cultures

How women from different cultures report different symptoms of menopause. Attitudes to age and sexuality in different cultures. How cultural forces and socio-economic status affect women's experience of – and attitude to – menopause. Results of recent research into cross-cultural experience of menopause.

There are two views about severity and frequency of menopausal symptoms. The view held by health professionals is that it is a biological transition in a woman's life that can be medically managed and treated by hormone therapy. The other view, held by feminists and social scientists, is that it is a natural phrase of a woman's life that is often culturally determined. Some women go through it unnoticed and without medication.

Menopause at mid-life can be a stressful time for some women. In addition to the normal physiological changes that our bodies are going through, it is usually a time when our lives are full of change: we must deal with our elderly parents, or with their loss, our children are leaving home, we face changes in our career, even the loss of a job. For others, this is the beginning of a new life. They are more at peace with themselves, feeling that they are their own person.

Women from different cultural and socio-economic backgrounds perceive and experience menopause differently and report a great difference in symptoms and their severity. These range from experiencing no discomfort to experiencing a multitude of symptoms. Factors contributing to these differences are women's socio-cultural and economic status, their educational background, personality, religious beliefs, and their diet and nutritional status.

In a recent comprehensive literature review entitled 'Menopause across culture', Helen Ryan (Mid-Link Menopause Service, 1999) compiled a summary of over sixty cross-cultural menopause studies conducted over the past forty years in Europe, North America, Africa and Australia. They show up the complexity of the interaction and the nexus between the physiological changes of menopause and the social and cultural components of women's lives.

The author points out that symptoms vary across cultures, with Asian women experiencing a lower frequency and severity of complaints compared to European/American women. Western culture can be youth-orientated and tags middle age as unattractive, unfashionable and unwanted. We just have to flick through the pages of magazines to be convinced of such views. But in non-western cultures there is less emphasis on glamour, youth and fashion, so women approaching menopause in those places feel less threatened and perceive this transitional phase more positively. No wonder these women report fewer menopausal problems than their western counterparts.

It appears that women's experiences of menopause can vary significantly within and across cultures, even though the age at which menopause occurs is fairly similar. By way of illustration, women in Asian, African, Middle East and South American countries experience menopausal symptoms differently when compared to women from Australian, American and European backgrounds. The former group neither perceives the symptoms as something to worry about nor complains about their menopausal problems. Cultural forces play an important role in women's perception and experience of menopause.

A woman's cultural background is made up of expectations, beliefs, religious views, dietary consumption and living conditions, literacy skills, and attitudes towards sexuality, reproduction and ageing. Often the differences in women's experiences of menopause can be attributed to the differences between and within cultures.

Although the results we read in the literature might be contradictory, there is not a significant difference in the physiological experiences in postmenopausal women from different cultures. But there is significant variation in psychological well-being and cultural beliefs about ageing. Asian women, for example, seldom report menopausal symptoms to their doctors, and they seem to suffer less frequently from depression than their western counterparts, although they suffer in the same way from osteoporosis and cardiovascular complications as the Caucasian women.

Women from western countries report symptoms of menopause, such as hot flushes, more frequently, and are said to experience them more severely. But women who seek medical advice for hot flushes are not the ones with the most severe symptoms. Western women are willing to take charge of their own health, and are more willing to discuss their symptoms with a medical practitioner, seek relief for their symptoms, search for competent providers and experiment with different therapies.

Australian women often say that they could not come to terms with menopause because it represented an invisible stepping-stone into old age; they saw the menopause as the end of their femininity and sexual attractiveness.

Although up to 70 per cent of Australian postmenopausal women report having hot flushes, studies conducted in Australia demonstrate a direct correlation between the rate of seeking help and stress-related issues. In other words, the women who were stressed found the symptoms of menopause difficult to tolerate.

In the Melbourne Women's Midlife Health Study, 2,000 randomly selected Australian-born women, aged between forty-five and fifty-five, were questioned about attitudes to menopause. Fewer menopausal symptoms, lower levels of stress, increased exercise participation and more positive attitudes to ageing and menopause were reported from women who had more years of education (Dennerstein *et al.*, 1993).

Similarly, American and Western European women perceive menopause as a medical condition and seek treatment more frequently. Oddens and Boulet in 1997 reported in *Obstetrics and Gynecology*, the results of a cross-sectional national survey of 1,015 Danish women aged between forty-five and sixty-five. Over 67 per cent of these women who had experienced menopausal complaints had consulted a physician, and about 30 per cent had used hormone replacement therapy to elevate climacteric symptoms.

In 1999 in the *Medical Journal of Australia* Alastair MacLennan and his colleagues reported that Australians are the biggest users of hormone replacement therapy in the world. A survey of 1,049 South Australian women showed that about 40 per cent of Australian women were using hormone replacement therapy around the age of menopause, with use in the fifty-five to sixty-four age bracket doubling since a similar study in 1991. About 60 per cent of women in this age group had used the therapy at some point.

Overall, Australian, American and British studies have shown that the socio-economic status and the level of education are directly related to the menopausal symptoms experienced and reported by women. They see menopause as a medical condition requiring treatment.

It appears that women from western cultures perhaps have higher health expectations. On the other hand, a small proportion of Eastern European women use hormone replacement therapy largely because they remain poorly informed about the therapy. Although the prevalence of postmenopausal symptoms is the same in Eastern Europe compared to Western Europe, according to studies, hormone replacement therapy is used by fewer people in Eastern Europe and the duration of therapy is shorter.

The signs of postmenopausal symptoms in Asian women are high, but the number of symptoms that they recognise as problems and complain about are low. They report hot flushes less frequently than women in the west and are unlikely to seek medical treatment for the menopause. In many Asian countries, women accept menopause as a matter of fact, as a natural transition in their life, and do not seek treatment for their symptoms. A study reported by Boulet *et al.* in 1994 was conducted in seven south-east Asian countries: Hong Kong, Indonesia, Korea, Malaysia, the Philippines, Singapore and Taiwan. Approximately 400 women were questioned in each country about a number of menopausal complaints. The data showed that although the symptoms were experienced in south-east Asian countries they were milder than those reported in the west and less prevalent.

> 'I think most Australian women have an expectation that certain things will start happening when they reach menopause because that's the norm. But in Asia we practically don't even know what it is.'
>
> JANNIE TAY

Observational studies of close to 400 women reported independently by two groups, Samil and Wishuwardhani (1994) and Ismael (1994), show that in countries such as Malaysia and Indonesia more than 70 per cent of the study population had no serious menopausal symptoms. Only 20 to 30 per cent of the women consulted a doctor about their menopausal symptoms and, of these, 84 per cent were given a prescription but 43 per cent did not take the medication.

Studies of Japanese women published by Lock in 1994 show that Asian women report significantly lower frequency of hot flushes compared to their North American counterparts but report different menopausal symptoms such as headaches, stiff shoulders and vaginal problems.

Studies by McCarthy in 1994 show Chinese women from Singapore and Hong Kong report hot flushes less frequently than western women, but that other symptoms such as irritability and insomnia were more frequently recorded. These women were also using hormone replacement therapy less frequently than the western women.

Often the medical attitude as well as the general perception of the community and society towards menopause and middle age will affect women's expectations of treatment.

Cultural influences appear to affect women's ability to tolerate menopausal symptoms because in some cultures it is considered healthy to suppress physiological and psychological symptoms. Recent cross-cultural studies reported in 1999 by Gabriella Berger of seventy Australian and seventy Filipino menopausal women living in Australia found no differences in physical menopause experiences between the Filipino and Australian women but a significant variation in terms of physiological well-being and cultural beliefs about ageing. Although most of the Filipino women were coping with menopausal symptoms, a quarter of the Australian women, who exhibited signs of depression, irritability and mood swings, said that they could not come to terms with menopause because it represented an inevitable stepping-stone into old age.

When comparing cross-cultural studies, we have to bear in mind that cultural differences affect the way women perceive, tolerate and experience menopausal symptoms. The richness of the language also has an effect when we try to compare menopausal symptoms across different cultures. There are no equivalent words for 'hot flush' in Japanese and Chinese or for 'menopause' in Japanese. And in Japan, menstruation and menopause are viewed differently from the way they are viewed in the west. Menarche in Japan is not only celebrated but also widely announced to family members. Although menopause is not announced and women lose their reproductive power, they gain a different respect, and feel more liberated socially and emotionally.

In other Asian countries, including China and Korea, there is a view that, through menopause and ageing, women gain respect from younger women.

As illustrated in Miriam Stoppard's book *Menopause*, in some traditional societies menopause signals increased social status and sexual liberation. As an illustration, the Maya postmenopausal women in Central America are said to appreciate the improved social status, renewed freedom, greater respect and power. The women become heads of extended families and are unlikely to seek medical help during menopause. In others, older women are regarded as equal to men and play an important decision-making role in the family.

In India, for example, postmenopausal women enjoy new freedom as they join the men for drinks and chat, walk freely and enjoy the respect of younger people, none of which was allowed before menopause. In addition, larger extended families means that younger women tend to do more labour-intensive tasks, thus allowing the postmenopausal women more time for themselves. In these women a wide range of views about menopause was expressed, and benefits such as being and feeling free have been noted.

Of the 405 postmenopausal Indian women interviewed for a study reported by Sharma and Saxena in *Maturatas* in 1981, the majority showed that they experienced their climacteric as very distressing, but only 10 per cent had sought medical treatment because menopause is still a taboo subject.

Observational studies indicate that women from African countries experience menopause differently. Zimbabwean women, for example, experience a loss in status, while for women in Botswana menopause confers a higher status.

It has been noted that in some developing countries, such as Africa and South America and in rural areas of Asian countries, women become menopausal at a younger age than the women in developed countries. Life expectancy also varies across cultures. In western countries, life expectancy is about eighty-two years, while in some underdeveloped countries women are expected to live to their mid fifties. For these women menopausal issues are less important compared to heart and other related diseases.

There has been an increasing trend in Asian countries of reporting menopausal symptoms due to an increased awareness of women's health and a greater understanding of women's perception of menopause. There is no doubt that the exposure to western culture is a contributing factor.

It appears that menopause is a cross-cultural experience and the environment, diet, activity patterns, fertility patterns and cultural values affect both the menopausal experience and the health of women as they age.

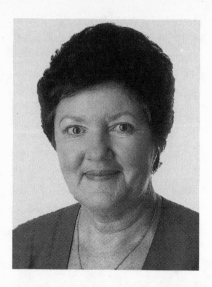

Joan Kirner, AM, was encouraged by her family to become well educated. She attended university, became a secondary school teacher and involved herself in community activities for over thirty-five years. While her children were young, she fought for a quality education for them and became involved in lobbying at local, state and national level for better standards of education. This experience led to her passion for participation and equity and her election to the Victorian Parliament. She held at various times in her parliamentary career the positions of Minister of Conservation, Minister for Education, and Minister for Women. In August 1990, Joan Kirner became the first female Premier of Victoria. Joan is proud to be a feminist. She is committed to equity, choice, diversity and advocacy for women and the community.

Joan Kirner

I have to say that I was always looking forward to menopause and the end of menstruation. I'd had my three children and I was hoping for an early menopause like my mother, who reached menopause in her late forties.

Around the time I was Minister for Education in the late eighties, I started to notice heavier flows. That was my main problem – coping with the potential for embarrassing situations.

And then, one day, the inevitable happened. I was addressing a deputation when the flooding occurred and I was wearing, of all things, a white suit. I passed a note to my adviser which said, 'Just get them out of here!' We politely got rid of them.

My friends told me to go and seek some help for the flooding, so I finally went to a gynaecologist and had a curette. By the time I had moved into the role of Premier, the symptoms had become a little more manageable, although I had always suffered from migraines around my periods. I did often wonder how Jeff Kennett would have coped with the same circumstances.

So really, I just basically managed at first. Then, towards the end of that period, I started experiencing the hot flushes and it all got a bit unmanageable. So I went off to a menopause clinic and found them really good to talk to. They checked me out, tested me for osteoporosis, the works.

I had hormone replacement patches for about six months, but my body felt too heavy while I was on it, and I think my psyche resented the intervention. A girlfriend, who's younger than me, was also having a few problems and her doctor put her on hormone replacement therapy too. She told me that they made no enquiries about her family history, nothing, before they prescribed it. I was horrified; her mother had actually died of cancer. I'd had everything checked out before I went on hormone replacement therapy, but I didn't persist.

I have always taken a vitamin B complex, and walked regularly in the mornings. This has always helped me keep up my energy. If I felt there was something else worth trying, I wouldn't have a problem with trying it.

I was lucky enough to avoid any drastic mood swings during menopause. Overall, I'm a fairly even-tempered person, and I've always held the view that moods are one thing that we need to keep in check and not impose on other people. This didn't change.

But I did suffer from fluid retention and, in the end, I really didn't realise just how tired I'd become. I saw myself on a television interview one night, and said to myself, It's time for a rethink. I looked so exhausted. And I was.

Then I did the inevitable. I tripped and broke a wrist, then I tripped again and had a compound fracture of the elbow. That pretty much confirmed that both Parliament and the premiership had taken their toll on my health.

I think I must have inherited my mother's strong genes and determination, so I simply carried on with my day-to-day commitments. If a job has to be done then there's not much sense cancelling an appointment simply because of heavy bleeding or a migraine. You just learn to cope.

I never really thought that the onset of menopause was a sign that I was growing old. It was simply something that you lived through while you got on with the real job. In fact, I feel more of that now. I have a lot more aches and pains than I ever used to.

Other than putting on weight, it was a relief to move beyond menopause and being the centre of public attention, especially when I could swap from high heels to flat shoes and casual gear again.

I don't follow any particular exercise regime and I don't have any special diet. I do go for regular walks with friends, but I think I probably need to look a bit more closely at the required diet and exercise, for a busy family and work life out of the limelight.

Really, the major effect on me at this time in my life has not been so much the menopause but the change from being in the political spotlight to being in the background. This has been quite a big period of personal and family readjustment.

When I left politics I received a lump sum payment but no parliamentary pension. The lump sum was not enough to provide for my old age; I needed another job. That was a bit of a shock at first. But Paul Keating offered me a full-time chair at the new Employment Authority and that was a great way to re-focus and still be an achiever.

Ron, my husband, and I bought a caravan in 1996 for travelling in the outback. I make more time for myself and for my grandchildren, as well as being the chair and committee member of several advisory boards.

These days, I try to live a more balanced life and focus my work activities building a new women's political support network called Emily's List which helps women trying to get into Parliament. We are having amazing success.

When I look back, I see my life has been divided into decades. While my principles have always remained the same, it seems that something different has happened in every decade that affected my direction. I see the decade from 1995 to 2005 as an opportunity to make an effective change for women in politics. I see my role now as similar to the way I saw other women some forty years ago, only today I am the mentor who can pass on my own experience to younger women. I feel that I'm helping to break new ground by creating networks with a different cultural view of politics and offering my support and advice as a role model to the next generation of Australian women politicians.

I have worked in life not necessarily to change the world but to change the little bit of the world where I and other feminists can make a difference. That's my passion, and it's my passion that keeps me going.

Chapter Three
Mood changes

Reasons for mood changes at midlife. Are women more likely to suffer depression in menopause? Is there such a thing as the 'empty nest syndrome'? What therapies are available. A definition of depression.

Women often report changes in mood at menopause. The psychological symptoms most noted are irritability, fatigue, difficulty in coping, depression and anxiety. Many are sleep deprived. They may be woken frequently at night by hot flushes and night sweats, and quite reasonably may feel irritable and tired.

Other factors that may have an effect on mood at this time of life include concerns about ageing, stressful events, physical illnesses and psychosocial issues. Women at menopause often have many stresses in their daily lives, which may include dealing with ageing parents, coping with adolescent children, financial difficulties, employment outside the home, and sometimes marital difficulties. Domestic abuse, childhood sexual abuse, and alcohol or drug abuse can increase the risk of depressive illness.

Women who are in paid employment often have greater self-esteem, whereas loss of a job or unemployment may lead to depression. Other losses may occur – for example, the death of parents, spouse, children or friends.

Confronting one's mortality through the perception that menopause is the beginning of old age may also predispose women to anxiety or depression or both.

Loss of reproductive capacity may strongly affect women who would have liked to have had more children, have been unable to have children, or have delayed having a family for various reasons until it is too late.

Although many women complain of mood changes in the perimenopausal years, and hormonal changes may contribute to the symptoms, moderate to severe depression is not more common at this stage of life than at other stages.

> 'I remember being enormously angry with everybody. Now I tend to accept my problems rather than lay blame elsewhere. After all, life is full of problems. But, back then, I always thought that my anger was connected to nearing menopause.'
>
> ITA BUTTROSE

Some studies of women who go to doctors or seek help at menopause clinics have found that depression is relatively more common among them than in the general community. This is not an unexpected observation, as women who have significant depressive symptoms at menopause in all probability will seek help. It might also be expected that they attribute their increase in depressive symptoms to the hormonal changes they are experiencing.

Depression is common in our society. About a fifth of the population is likely to experience a significant depressive illness at some stage in their life. It is probably under-diagnosed and therefore under-treated in many people. Among those who commit suicide, many have not been diagnosed with depression or have not been considered by their relatives or friends to be depressed. Suicide is the cause of death in 15 per cent of depressed people, and depression recurs in up to 80 per cent of people who have one initial depressive illness.

Certain socio-economic and psychological factors are the main predictors for depression in women at menopause. These include a past history of depression, lower socio-economic status, stressful life events and chronic ill health. Other factors that may predispose them to depression include unemployment, marital status, that is, being separated or divorced, having a lack of social support, having a surgical menopause, and holding negative beliefs about menopause.

'Mood swings certainly affected me. But in my case, if I was feeling out of sorts, or that the world was against me, or that nothing I was doing was right, then I just got on and got busy with something. It was the best cure I knew.'

TONIA TODMAN

Mid-life is often characterised by negative thoughts about ageing. And in our society negative attitudes are often held towards women at menopause, particularly in western societies, which tend to focus on youth and beauty as desirable feminine qualities compared with age, wisdom and experience.

One of the myths put forward as a predisposing factor to depression at menopause is the 'empty nest syndrome'. There is a belief that women grieve for their children who have left home to study or work. A study in the US, which found that women whose children had left home had 'greater happiness, greater enjoyment of life, and greater marital harmony' than women who still had children at home, has dispelled this myth.

Some women appear to be particularly sensitive to hormonal changes throughout life so that those women who have suffered from severe psychological premenstrual symptoms and significant post-natal depression, particularly if it lasted for more than six weeks, may be at risk of depression recurring at menopause.

Some studies on depression in postmenopausal women have shown that oestrogen replacement therapy may be of help. Other studies have not shown a benefit. Some studies have demonstrated good results from higher than standard doses of hormone replacement therapy.

If there are significant physical symptoms, such as hot flushes, and depressive symptoms, hormone replacement therapy should be tried. There are other more specific therapies known to be effective in the treatment of depression, which may be added if the depressive symptoms persist despite adequate doses of hormone replacement therapy.

Many women who suffer depression are reluctant to seek help, and often very reluctant to consider antidepressant therapy. They feel that they are a failure for not being able to overcome their depressive feelings themselves. There is unfortunately still a stigma in our community about psychological and psychiatric illness. Poorly informed people often hold these prejudices.

Many mental illnesses have a genetic and biochemical basis or tendency. As with many physical illnesses, this predisposition is influenced by environmental factors, particularly stressful life events. In women, hormonal changes during reproductive life can also contribute to the expression of this underlying susceptibility.

A simple explanation of depression is helpful. There is a relationship between hormonal and biochemical changes in the brain and depression. It allows many women to accept and be comfortable with using antidepressive treatment and enables them to overcome their often-incapacitating illness and to resume a normal life.

Other than hormone replacement therapy, there are several treatments available for treating depression and anxiety symptoms. The most commonly used group of relatively new therapies is the serotonin uptake inhibitors, known as the SSRIs.

Serotonin is what we call a 'neurotransmitter'. It is a vital biochemical substance involved in the nerve pathways within the brain that are related to pain perception, mood and sleep. Low oestrogen levels have been shown to be associated with lower serotonin levels in the brain. As a result, musculoskeletal aches and pains, mild depression and poor sleeping patterns are very common symptoms in menopausal women. The SSRIs are even more effective than oestrogen in improving serotonin levels.

The commonly used brand names for these SSRIs are Prozac (fluoxetine), Zoloft (sertraline), Aropax (paroxtetine) and Luvox (fluovoxamine). They are all effective, but individuals may have a more favourable response and fewer side effects with one drug rather than another. Clinical trials have found that some of these drugs are effective in treating premenstrual symptoms and postnatal depression.

Two other neurotransmitters in particular are implicated in depression. They are noradrenaline and dopamine. Serotonin and noradrenaline are biochemical substances that are influenced by other drugs with similar actions to the SSRIs. They are called SNRIs. Two commonly prescribed drugs in this group are Serzone (nefazadone) and Efexor (venlafaxine).

'I'd say I have recently been through ten really tough years, and I do feel a sense of release at having dealt with them. I got through them. I can relax now feeling that I am in control of my own destiny.'

STEPHANIE ALEXANDER

Common side effects of the SSRIs and the SNRIs include nausea, headache, insomnia, agitation and sexual dysfunction – in particular, reduced libido. They are less sedating and in general there is less weight gain. SSRIs and SNRIs do not have the toxic effect on the heart that other antidepressants may have in overdosage.

An older group of drugs collectively called 'tricyclic' antidepressives or TCAs are sometimes still prescribed. In low doses, they can be helpful for chronic pain management, such as in fibromyalgia, but they can cause significant side effects particularly if overdosage occurs. They cause dry mouth, affect memory and concentration, and are not well tolerated by older women. They have, however, been used for postnatal depression and have been shown to be safe in this situation.

Some women will not be able to tolerate any of these drugs and may find benefit from some of the much older drugs that have been used for depression. These medications are used less commonly these days because of side effects or potentially adverse interactions with other drugs or foods.

Menopause occurs at a time in life when women may be experiencing many changes and stresses, such as separations, relationship difficulties with partners, parents and adolescents. They may have concerns about ageing and a feeling of rejection by a society that favours youth and wrinkle-free beauty. But many women see positive opportunities opening up for them at midlife, so that with any luck menopause for them is just a phase that they pass through and adjust to, as they may have needed to adjust during other stages of their lives.

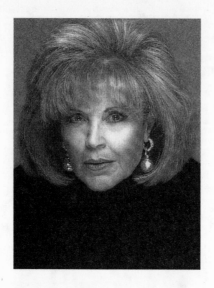

Lillian Frank, AM, MBE, was born in
Rangoon, Burma. Lillian has been a public and
media personality for many years. At different times
in her colourful career she has worked as a society
hairdresser, radio commentator, TV personality and
columnist (she writes a weekly column for the
Melbourne *Herald-Sun*). Known for her dynamism
and frenetic pace, she has always been active in
cultural, charity, educational and sporting enterprises. She is, for example, a Life Governor of the
Royal Children's and the Royal Women's Hospitals,
Chairman of the Special Events Committee for the
Royal Children's Hospital, a patron of Odyssey
House for mentally retarded minors, an ambassador
for MBMC, Australia Day, and the International
World Cup Tournament, a former board member of
the Opera Foundation of Victoria, Foundation
Patron of Richmond West Primary School, Patron
of Dandenong Valley Special development School,
Chair of the VRC Derby Eve Committee and a
member of Friends of Peter McCallum Hospital.

Lillian Frank

Menopause is a fact of life. It's evolution. You're born. You don't ask to be born, but suddenly you're there, and from then on you go through the evolution of life.

Every year in your life is a bonus; it doesn't matter whether you are old or young. You get up in the morning and you are lucky to be alive, lucky to be doing the things you like doing in your life. You take the bat and ball and keep playing. That's what life is all about.

If I had any discomfort during menopause, I tended to simply cope with it the same as I did with the rest of life's challenges. A lot of my friends often get lonely, or sad, or they have nothing to do. Believe it or not, this happens to a lot of women with very comfortable homes and very wealthy husbands. They often suffer more from these things because they tend to make mountains out of molehills. On the other hand, busy people who are racing around with the demands of their lives don't have time to dwell on their aches and pains.

I didn't feel the need for any medication. I don't like to take tablets, not for a headache or anything. I need to be dying before I take a pain killer. I believe that the pain or sickness is a result of something I've done to temporarily muck up my system – I was in a hurry or didn't eat breakfast, something like that. The pain won't be there forever, and it's not going to kill me, so I just cope with the discomfort until it passes. I don't believe in putting just anything down my throat.

At one stage during my menopause, I went to a male doctor who was terribly patronising. I had come to see him because I was very worried about my breasts, which had become quite large, and I was having headaches. Although I wasn't suffering too much, I thought I would have a check-up. But the doctor just carried on about how wonderful it was to be advising a celebrity, and all this business.

I said, 'Look, I'm not here as a celebrity. I'm here merely as a woman who wants some help.'

He asked me a lot of questions, gave me some tablets and told me to ring him if there were any problems.

Now, I'm the sort of person who sticks to my word. If I tell you to ring me and I'm not available, then I'll ring you back as soon as I am available. I rang this doctor five times, and each time his nurse said he was busy and he would ring me back. Five days later, when he finally rang me, I said, 'Thank you, but you're five days too late.' I'm not going to be mucked around by a man when I need help.

So I went to a woman doctor who was absolutely fantastic. After a few weeks of medication that didn't help at all, she threw my tablets in the rubbish bin and put me on vitamins. I've been taking calcium, vitamin E and vitamin C ever since and I've never looked back.

I've always been a very healthy person. I've only had two operations in my life. One was to remove my appendix, which I had in India when I was about eight. It was a disaster. The other was a thyroid operation two years ago. Apart from those, I've had no problems. I've been very lucky.

I might be getting older, but I haven't got time to worry about every line on my face. Although I don't drink, I do love my food, and I eat a lot. But now I've learnt to eat in a different way.

I've been through just about every diet in the world. All this nonsense about two pounds less or two pounds more just doesn't help. What you need to do is have a good hard look at yourself and see what makes you fat and decide to do something serious about it. You need a strong mental attitude, and you must read books to educate yourself about the right things to do.

I've got my own eating regime now. My daughter, Jackie, editor of *Marie Claire*, reads a lot, and she suggested that I eat a moderate amount of carbohydrates for lunch, protein for dinner and cut out all fats. I still follow that diet.

Going out is a big part of my job and my way of life. When I go out, I'm very careful with what I eat. If it's a function in a big hotel, for example, I'll make sure that I can get a salad or fish or something like that. At a restaurant, you have more choice, but when you go to a hotel function you need to be more prepared.

Over the next twenty years, my health will be my first priority. I don't drink and I don't smoke, not because I'm a good person or anything like that. I do all sorts of funny things that nobody else would do, but I can't see any reason for drinking. It doesn't give me any pleasure. I like to focus on the things that give me, and others, pleasure.

I also go to the gymnasium three times a week. Even though my time is precious, I still get up at 7.30 and go there. I have a trainer for motivation and for help with my exercises, and he is absolutely fabulous. He's also a physiotherapist and a fitness fanatic. He pushes me to the limit, and then I go over the limit with him.

As you get older, I think is important to have regular check-ups with your doctor. It's something you have to do, and you would be foolish not to. A lot of people say they are frightened of the doctor, but I believe you should make the effort to find one you trust and see them regularly.

I don't believe in alternative medicines. I know a lot of people believe in them, but I'm very strong-minded, and I think it's all in the head. I was once at a show that featured a hypnotist, and I was called up on stage to be a subject. Well, I knew it wouldn't work on me, and I even had a bet with my friend to prove it so. After a while the hypnotist asked me to return to the audience – he had a big audience, and I was making it bad for him. I remember he said, 'Well that's one person you can't do anything about.' I guess I feel the same way about alternative medicines.

As far as activities go, I'm still doing everything I've done for the past twenty years. I think you are either one of those people who wants to keep doing things or you're a person who feels constrained by the changes in your life.

I don't have to re-evaluate my life just because I'm getting older. I'm probably doing more now than before because, as my life has changed, opportunities have come my way. I'm not the sort of person who just comes for the ride. If I take something on, then I'm there for the long haul.

Chapter Four
Hormone replacement therapy

Overview of hormone replacement therapy, how it has changed over the years, the role of oestrogen and progestins. How hormone replacement therapy relieves the symptoms of menopause, and its benefits for bone strength. Risks of taking hormone replacement therapy: does it increase the risk of breast cancer? does it cause weight gain? risks of blood clots in the lungs and Alzheimer's. Types of hormone replacement therapy available and how they are administered. Side effects of hormone replacement therapy.

One of the controversial issues for women is whether they should use hormone replacement therapy. Menopause is a natural event in women's lives, and many critics of hormone therapy treatment consider that using hormone therapy is an example of over medicalisation of a normal physiological process. This argument is not unique to menopause. Similar criticism is put forward about infertility treatment, contraception, pregnancy and childbirth and the medical care of elderly women.

The debate is always being brought into the public awareness by reports in the media of the possible cancer-causing effects of hormone replacement therapy, particularly the possible increased risk of breast cancer.

Hormone replacement has been used for many years. Initially it was used in the United States with just oestrogen. After some years of oestrogen use, it was noted that there was an increase in the rate of endometrial cancer, or cancer of the lining of the uterus. There is a dose-related effect on the risk of endometrial cancer, as well as an effect with longer use. In other words, the higher the dose of oestrogen and the longer it is taken the greater the effect that it has on the endometrium and the greater the likelihood of developing endometrial cancer.

The risk of developing endometrial cancer is reduced significantly if progestins are added to the therapy. Progestin therapy should be taken for twelve to fourteen days each month if cyclical therapy is used, or continuously if you wish to avoid having a withdrawal bleed. A withdrawal bleed is bleeding that occurs one to two days after stopping the course of progestin.

Older women do not need to have a withdrawal bleed if the hormones are given in balanced doses. In women who are only one to two years beyond their menopause it is usually preferable to give intermittent or monthly progestin therapy as the lining of the uterus is thicker and irregular bleeding is more common. Shorter use of progestins – that is, for fewer than twelve days – may not adequately protect the lining from abnormal changes.

A small number of women are unable to tolerate any of the available progestin therapies but still need to use oestrogen to control menopausal symptoms. These women may decide to use oestrogen alone and have the lining of the uterus sampled every year to assess whether any abnormal changes are developing.

Newer therapies, incorporating progestins, are being evaluated, and they may suit some women who cannot tolerate oral progestins. One such treatment is an intrauterine device containing a progestin called levonorgestrel (marketed as Mirena). It is also used as a form of contraception in premenopausal women. Oestrogen plus progestin patches are also available now. Ooestrogen is used for fourteen days followed by fourteen days of oestrogen plus progestin patches (called cyclical therapy), or oestrogen plus progestin patches are used continuously throughout the whole month (called continuous therapy). As the dose of progestin is lower than in oral therapy it may be less likely to produce adverse side effects.

The common symptoms reported by women around menopause are hot flushes, sweats, anxiety, vaginal dryness, depression, painful intercourse, irritability, headaches, poor memory, sexual dysfunction, loss of libido, palpitations, poor concentration, dizzy spells, sleeplessness, muscle/joint pains, and dry, itchy skin. Many of these symptoms will respond to oestrogen and oestrogen/progestin replacement therapy.

Most women will be helped by using hormone replacement therapy for their hot flushes and sweats, although not all women will need or want to take it. Hormone replacement therapy can improve quality of life if symptoms are considered to be affecting it. But it is not a panacea for treating all the symptoms or health concerns of women at menopause. The decision should be an individual one and taken only after all the benefits and risks have been discussed with a doctor.

'My doctor explained that there was no such thing as a Fountain of Youth, but hormone replacement therapy was the next best thing. I must say, I haven't missed a beat.'

JEANNE PRATT

During the perimenopausal years, hormone levels and the menstrual cycle may vary. If there are symptoms, such as hot flushes, but periods are still relatively frequent, one of the low-dose oral contraceptive pills may provide good cycle control and relief of symptoms.

If you are uncertain about the benefits of either the oral contraceptive pill or hormone replacement therapy for your symptoms, then a two- to three-month trial of therapy can be used. Starting and stopping is not a problem. Unlike other medications, hormone replacement therapy is not an essential treatment. Women who have significant symptoms, however, are usually very grateful that there is a treatment that can help them.

Mild depressive symptoms can be helped with hormone replacement use, but moderate to severe depression will usually need antidepressant medication. Young women who have had their ovaries removed may respond to both oestrogen and testosterone replacement therapy, but some need only oestrogen. Some older postmenopausal women may also want to try testosterone therapy as well as oestrogen therapy if they are troubled by a reduced sex drive.

Hormone replacement therapy can have a positive effect on bone mass – an important issue for older women. Oestrogen increases bone density. In observational studies comparing hormone replacement therapy users with non-hormone replacement therapy users, oestrogen has been reported to reduce spinal and hip fractures. But there are no randomised, controlled trials that have reported the effects of oestrogen in reducing hip fractures, and only one or two short-term randomised controlled studies have shown a reduction in spinal fractures.

'[My doctor] got very cross with me and said, "I suppose you're the sort of woman that wouldn't take HRT if you didn't want to." And I said, "That's right." I'm of the view that my body is mine and if I don't wish to put anything into it, nobody can make me.'

ITA BUTTROSE

There are a range of medications (as discussed in the chapter on osteoporosis) that have been shown in randomised, controlled trials to reduce spinal fractures. The bisphosphonate group of drugs, which are used for osteoporosis, have been shown in randomised, controlled clinical trials to reduce spinal and hip fractures. The two drugs that have been shown to be beneficial for both types of fracture are alendronate (marketed as Fosamax) and risedronate (marketed as Actonel). Another type of medication that has an oestrogen-like effect on bone, called raloxifene (marketed as Evista), has also been shown in randomised, controlled trials to reduce spinal fractures. They would be suitable in the treatment of osteoporosis in women who cannot take hormone replacement therapy, such as those women who have had a past history of breast cancer.

The two most common reasons that women give for feeling anxious about using hormone replacement are the risk of weight gain and the risk of developing breast cancer.

Breast cancer is a common cancer in postmenopausal women for which the most significant risk factor is increasing age. A family history of breast cancer in first-degree relatives – that is, sister, mother and daughter – particularly if it occurs premenopausally – is also a strong risk factor.

There are many other factors that have been implicated in increasing the risk of breast cancer by a small degree. One of these is long-term exposure to oestrogen. This long-standing exposure may be due to an early menarche (starting periods early) or to a late menopause. Women who have an early or premature menopause appear to have a reduced risk of breast cancer.

A controversial question about hormone replacement is whether taking oestrogen for five, ten, fifteen years or longer after the age of fifty will increase the risk of breast cancer. In the chapter on breast disease some of the recent studies are discussed.

A study reported in the *Lancet* in 1997 re-analysed 90 per cent of the world's epidemiological information on the relationship between hormone replacement therapy and breast cancer. Longer durations of recent use, but not past use of hormone replacement therapy (oestrogen alone and oestrogen/progestin therapies) increased the risk of breast cancer, particularly in leaner women.

An editorial in the same issue of the journal commented on the results of the study. They predicted that the risk of breast cancer increased to 80 per cent after ten years' use and 120 per cent after twenty years' use. Although these figures seem to show a huge increase in the risk of getting breast cancer as a result of using hormone replacement therapy, the risk is really relatively small compared with the risk brought about by a woman's increasing age.

Women who have been on long-term hormone therapy for prevention of heart disease and osteoporosis need to weigh up their risk of using hormone replacement therapy in this way as well as considering any other risk factors they may have for breast cancer. In these studies short-term use of hormone replacement therapy, for five years or less, for example, has not been shown to increase the risk of getting breast cancer.

As far as the prevention of heart disease is concerned, modifications in the way you live can be effective. There are also specific treatments, such as those to lower blood pressure and cholesterol levels.

The issue of hormone replacement therapy and weight gain has been of concern to many women. In many studies, it has been shown that, in general, perimenopausal and postmenopausal women, whether on hormone replacement therapy or not, have a tendency to gain weight. Overall, hormone replacement therapy may reduce the amount of weight gained. One possible mechanism is that women feel better on the medication and therefore are more motivated to exercise.

There is information from epidemiological studies that hormone replacement therapy use is associated with a small increase in the risk of pulmonary embolus (blood clots in the lung). The incidence of pulmonary embolus, however, is very small – about 1 in 5,000. Women who have had a spontaneous blood clot in their legs or have a strong family history of blood clots should seek specialist advice before taking hormone replacement therapy.

Although having had breast cancer is usually a reason to avoid using hormone replacement therapy, some women may decide that their quality of life is poor as a result of severe menopausal symptoms. These women need to be well informed about the risks before they decide to take hormone replacement therapy.

Other contraindications include cancer of the endometrium, a significant blood-clotting (thrombotic) tendency, and severe liver and kidney disease. There is a small increase in the incidence of gall bladder disease in women who use hormone replacement therapy. Any abnormal bleeding should always be investigated

Many women wonder if hormone replacement therapy may reduce their risk of developing Alzheimer's disease, particularly those who have a strong family history of it. They may have noticed a problem with their short-term memory around menopause and be worried that they may be developing Alzheimer's disease.

Oestrogen does play a role in the transmission of nerve pulses in the brain and the alteration of oestrogen levels can have a temporary effect on memory in some women. This effect is generally very minor. Other factors probably play a role in apparent problems with short-term memory at menopause.

Many women suffer from poor sleep and fatigue as a secondary effect of night sweats and hot flushes. They often find that their concentration is affected. Other stressful events in the daily lives of women can mean that their brains suffer 'information overload' and small issues may be easily forgotten. There is also a natural decline in memory as we all age, so that in most cases of memory problems there is definitely no indication that Alzheimer's disease is present.

There are many different oestrogen and progestin medications available. There are also many combinations of therapies and doses. Generally the standard dose is used – for example, the equivalent of 0.625 mg daily of Premarin as the oestrogen, and 10 mg of Provera for twelve to fourteen days or 5 mg continuously. Some formulations suit some women better than others, which is why there is such a variety.

Usually oral therapy is used and is acceptable to most women. Women who have problems with absorption may respond better to patches. Some women find that the higher blood levels achieved with oestrogen implants (sometimes with a testosterone implant as well) give more predictable symptom relief.

There are some differences in the effects of oral oestrogens and patches on cholesterol and tryglyceride levels. In general, these effects may not be important, except if there is a particular health problem. Women with high tryglyceride levels, for example, may be better using a patch form of oestrogen which doesn't increase tryglyceride levels.

There are many hormone replacement therapy regimes. Women who have had a hysterectomy can use continuous oestrogen orally, in patches or gels, or as implants. Women who still have their uterus can use continuous oestrogen (orally, in patches or gels, or as implants) combined with progestins either cyclically (12–14 days) or continuously.

Women who have vaginal dryness or bladder problems can use local oestrogen rings, pessaries, tablets or creams. These can be used with or without hormone replacement (that is, oral or patch forms of HRT), which have a general effect on the rest of the body.

Women who have sexual dysfunction or young women who have had their ovaries removed may add testosterone as oral, injection, patch or implant treatment in conjunction with their oestrogen treatment of choice.

All postmenopausal women on hormone replacement therapy should have regular check-ups. Six-monthly blood pressure and breast examinations and any others that are indicated by symptoms are desirable. Generally, at least yearly pap smears and yearly mammograms are recommended.

'When they brought out the patch I went straight on to it and have been using it now for over nine years. The stabilising effect was wonderful.'

DIANA ABRUZZI

The common side effects of hormone replacement therapy are fluid retention, breast enlargement and tenderness, nausea and headaches if you are on oestrogen treatment.

Premenstrual syndrome, depression, irritability, mood swings, bloating and headaches may occur if you are on progestins.

Irregular bleeding or heavy withdrawal bleeding may result from too low a dose or too high a dose of one hormone compared to the other. Generally a withdrawal bleed occurs one to two days after the course of progestin in cyclical treatment.

Breakthrough bleeding, when spotting or bleeding occurs erratically, can occur for up to six months with continuous use of progestin with oestrogen. If adjusting the dose doesn't settle the problem, or if the bleeding is clearly not what would be expected, further investigation is needed. This may involve a general and pelvic medical examination, a pap smear, a pelvic or vaginal ultrasound, or a hysteroscopy and curette. A hysteroscopy is a procedure whereby a long thin instrument with a tiny camera attached is inserted into the internal cavity of the uterus. Abnormalities that may be present can be transmitted and viewed on a video screen. A curette is a procedure whereby an instrument is guided gently but blindly into the cavity of the uterus and the lining is scraped away. A hysteroscopy is the best way of checking for the cause of abnormal bleeding.

The side effects of hormone replacement treatment can be avoided or improved by tailoring the dose to suit the woman. In older postmenopausal women who have not had hormone replacement therapy for many years or are many years postmenopausal, for example, starting with very small doses is important. The dose can then be built up gradually over a few months to avoid side effects. Young women, that is, women in their twenties or thirties may feel happier on much larger doses of hormones.

The metabolism and tolerance levels can vary widely, and what may be too much for one woman may be insufficient for another. Hormone levels are not routinely measured in women on oral therapy because the oestrogens are metabolised to a form that is not routinely measured by laboratories. Levels can be measured when women are on patches or implants because they contain oestradiol, which is the same hormone produced by the ovary and is the usual one measured in laboratories.

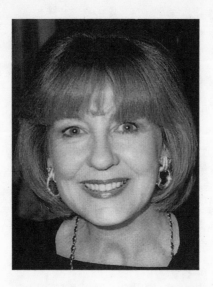

Elaine Canty has worked as a solicitor, a university tutor in clinical legal education and as a teacher of senior mathematics in London, but she is best known for her pioneering work and versatility in the media and sport. She was the first female sports broadcaster on ABC radio and television in Victoria and, in 1996, was the first woman to be appointed to the Australian Football League (AFL) Tribunal. Elaine presented a daily current affairs and talkback program on ABC radio 3LO for eight years and has covered three Olympic Games, anchoring the ABC broadcasts of the Barcelona Games. She runs Canty Communications Pty Ltd and makes frequent guest appearances and presentations for ABC radio and television. Outside her media work, she is a board member of VicHealth, the Women's and Children's Health Network, the Austin Research Institute, Athletics Australia and is a founding director of the Victoria Institute of Sport. She is married to the sports journalist Roy Masters and has three children.

Elaine Canty

I guess menopause just slid by me in many ways because the changes
coincided with so many other turbulent changes taking place in my
life such as remarriage, new career directions and the busy and
complex demands of family life with adult children.

Certainly I have had 'down' days and hormones may have had a
bit to do with that, but overwhelmingly I have a very happy life.

I'm very fortunate to have an extremely supportive family. My
parents, now in their eighties, are still astute and involved, and I have
three sisters and a brother. I am close to them all. I talk a lot to my
older sister about going through menopause.

I also have a tremendous group of girlfriends and we talk about
these things together very easily – I mean, we laugh about them.
When people close to you are going through the same experiences,
you don't feel so different, alienated or depressed. You start to wait for
the changes that others have already told you about. Then, if you do
experience any symptoms, they don't seem so bad, because you were
expecting the worst. And if you don't get any symptoms, you think,
Well aren't I lucky?

The one thing that has had an impact on me during menopause
was weight gain. I've always been very conscious of the way I look
because it's been very important to my work. Often I was the only

woman in a very male-dominated industry. I felt I had to be conscious of the way I looked because, as the only female, I attracted a fair amount of attention.

The weight gain bothered me a lot. I'm certainly heavier than I was ten years ago and that makes a difference to the way I feel about myself. I'm still conscious of my weight and appearance all the time. But when you're basically pretty happy with life, it's hard to find the incentive to really do something about the extra kilos. My husband is no help. He claims that in his eyes I am as gorgeous as ever.

I still keep physically active and enjoy things like cycling and trekking holidays, but I don't have as much energy as I used to.

I think that if I could lose another five or six kilos I'd feel more comfortable with myself, but I do find losing weight difficult. I especially like to sit down and relax at the end of the day over a glass of wine with my family. Giving up alcohol is hard because it represents something I enjoy very much in my life. I don't smoke or have any other vices, but I love my evening ritual.

Twice a week at 6.30 in the morning I meet a friend at the gym and we exercise for an hour and then have breakfast. I've been doing this for some years now, although with early morning work commitments I miss more of these morning sessions than I would like. But it is good discipline and the only really regular one I have.

I do a lot of walking. I'm trying to take up golf again, and I've resumed playing tennis because we have a court in the country. I've noticed lately that I'm nowhere near the agile tennis player I used to be. Nowadays, I'm relying heavily on cunning at the net and a hard serve.

I do try to watch my fat intake because I never feel as good when I've had fatty foods. I have to force myself to eat more fruit. While I quite like fruit, I'm not the sort of person that goes to the fridge and gets out an apple but I'm forcing myself to do that more consciously. I drink only skim milk now. I'm a meat eater, but if I go out I mostly eat fish or vegetables. We eat simply with a lot of lean meat and salad, lots of pasta dishes and fresh bread. My two absolute weaknesses are jam and fruit jelly. I'm also consciously drinking more water.

I'm sure I've felt more tired in recent times and I put that down to the extra weight. In fact, I blame everything on weight when maybe I should be blaming it on hormones. The tiredness could certainly be related to changes in my physiology, but, then again, when the day starts early and I'm always on the go, life in general is very demanding. Up until a couple of months ago I still had two children living permanently at home, and you find yourself very much involved in their lives as well as your own.

Now I find that people are beginning to see me as an 'older' woman when it doesn't seem all that long ago that I thought of myself simply as an attractive woman. This transition seems to have happened pretty fast for me – although for observers it probably hasn't happened quite so fast at all. I find it interesting that while I am now considered an older woman by men my own age and older, all of a sudden these men also seem older too. I'm now often working with men that are my age and older and it's very comfortable. Basically, I still feel like an attractive woman.

I was not unhappy to see the end of my monthly cycle. I used to suffer a lot from PMT, cramps, pain and the emotional ups and downs that go with your monthly period. Periods really governed my month because they were quite long and I had significant pain associated with them.

In some ways my period was like a welcome stranger because when it arrived it provided the reason for any mood swings and I'd think, Thank goodness it was my period and I'm not really going around the twist.

One change I have really noticed is in my joints. I am an extremely healthy person, but I have always had trouble with my knees, and now they are inclined to swell up after reasonably strenuous exercise. As my mother puts it – she's semi-disabled and walks with the aid of two sticks – 'The chassis is cracking up but the engine is running beautifully.'

I like to make the most of my physical health now because undoubtedly it will degenerate as I get older. I had to give up skiing some years ago because of injury, and I can't keep up the ten-hour days of trekking in the mountains like I used to. On a recent trekking trip to Patagonia, my knees blew up like balloons, and at the end of the day every step was agony. On our last trip we went to Cuba and I tried cycling. Now I've discovered cycling, it's terrific.

My working life has been very flexible and full of variety since I finished at 3LO. I go back from time to time to do a little bit of broadcasting. I like it that way. Everyone is pleased to see you go again.

I run a communication consultancy specialising in corporate training programs, and I have a busy public speaking schedule. I sit on quite a few boards and, as a result, a significant part of my working week is spent around meeting tables. I am also involved in a voluntary capacity in a number of sports and health organisations. I call it community service.

At this stage in life, I cherish times that I spend with people who matter. A friend of mine said to me the other day that you have to distinguish between what's urgent and what's important in your day.

I have no burning ambitions because life is rich with unexpected adventures. I have been fortunate to have travelled a lot. The more you travel and the more you do in your life, the more you appreciate the good things that you have. I would like to spend the next twenty years appreciating these good things.

Maybe I didn't realise this until I looked around me and saw that other people don't have what I've got. I'm not talking about material things. I've been very fortunate with my family. I have an extra-ordinarily interesting and loving husband – I am very close to my three children who have all reached adulthood without too much angst. I am extremely proud of them as fine human beings. My daughter is a secondary school teacher, one of my sons is a doctor and the other is doing final-year medicine.

I don't want to sound like a Pollyanna. Life has not always been as fulfilling and content as it is for me now. I had a dark stage in my forties going through the painful process of separation and divorce from my former husband after a long marriage. Around the same time I was undergoing major knee surgery, there was turmoil in management at my workplace and Mum was very ill. Fortunately life turned around before I had to think about dealing with the onset of menopause.

Chapter Five
Alternative therapies and supplements

Are there any alternative therapies to relieve symptoms of menopause? Phytoestrogens: how they work, the recent studies into their effectiveness, their role in the prevention of cardiovascular disease and osteoporosis. Chinese herbs, herbal teas, creams. The importance of various vitamins and which foods contain them. Minerals, particularly calcium, and how to reduce the loss of bone mass. Relaxation and exercise to relieve symptoms of stress.

It has been shown that about 50 per cent of western postmenopausal women undergo dietary changes to enhance their health at menopause. Various dietary modifications and supplements are used, such as phytoestrogens, antioxidants and essential fatty acids enriched diets. In addition, Chinese traditional medicine has gained popularity in relieving postmenopausal symptoms, and the use of various herbs, relaxation techniques, exercise and meditation are popular means of alternative health.

An Australian population survey of 3,000 people revealed that about half of those interviewed used at least one non-medically prescribed alternative or complementary medicine preparation. It is estimated that Australians spend more than $600 million per year on alternative therapies. According to 1997 Australian statistics, the alternative therapy industry in this country just a few years ago was worth more than $1 billion.

Of the alternative products that claim benefits on menopausal symptoms, only a few have been supported by scientific studies. A comprehensive review published in *Clinical Endocrinology and Metabolism* (Murkies *et al.*, 1998) and two articles written independently by Rachel Sharp and Laurie Howes in the *Medical Observer* in 1999 indicate that there is little doubt among the medical experts that alternative therapy can alleviate the number and severity of hot flushes experienced by postmenopausal women, but there is no conclusive evidence about the protection provided against osteoporosis and cardiovascular disease.

Some women will use both alternative therapies and conventional hormone replacement therapy to control their symptoms. One of the most popular alternative therapies are the phytoestrogens.

'I went to a woman doctor who was absolutely fantastic. After a few weeks of medication that didn't help at all, she threw my tablets in the rubbish bin and put me on vitamins. I've never looked back.'

LILLIAN FRANK

'Phyto' is a Greek word which means plant. Phytoestrogens are plant compounds with structures similar to that of oestrogen and therefore the body accepts them as oestrogens. But they are not as strong as naturally produced oestrogens or as potent as the oestrogen used in hormone replacement therapy preparations.

Over the last few years there has been an increasing interest in the role of phytoestrogens taken as dietary supplements in the treatment of menopausal symptoms. Phytoestrogens are used as alternative preparations to conventional hormone replacement therapy by perimenopausal and postmenopausal women who are either poorly tolerating the preparations of hormone replacement therapy or unwilling to take them for fear of an increased risk of breast cancer or other side effects.

If taken in high enough concentrations phytoestrogens, which are oestrogen-like naturally occurring substances, may provide an alternative source of oestrogen for women approaching menopause whose natural oestrogen production is in decline.

The main types of phytoestrogens are isoflavones, lignans and coumestans. Isoflavones, the most potent ones, are found in high concentrations in soya beans, red clovers, lentils, various varieties of beans, alfalfa sprouts and chickpeas. The principal isoflavones are genistein, daidzein and equol. This plant hormone has been studied most. Lignans and coumestrans are found in cereals, vegetables and particularly in linseed oil.

Once consumed in food, isoflavones are easily absorbed from the human gut into the bloodstream and are further processed in the liver, producing the active compounds genistein and daidzein. The microorganisms found in the gut as part of normal flora can also process isoflavones to produce active compounds, high levels of which can be measured in the urine and blood about five hours after eating isoflavone-rich food.

Different plant oestrogens have different potencies. For comparison, if oestradiol has a potency of 100, then genistein has a relative potency of 0.084, diadzein 0.013 and equol 0.061. The bioactivity of isoflavones, however, is similar to oestradiol when used at sufficiently high concentrations to produce a response.

Although a large percentage of western women complain about discomfort during menopause, most Asian women go through this phase of life with fewer reported menopausal symptoms. This may be due to cultural differences in the way women express postmenopausal symptoms. As we have seen, women from Asia, particularly Japan, are reported to have a lower incidence of hot flushes – about 5 per cent – compared to women in Europe and North America, where up to 70 per cent are reported to experience these symptoms.

Diet may account for some of it. The traditional Asian diet is rich in phytoestrogens. On average, women in the east consume between 30 and 80 mg of isoflavones each day, with the Japanese diet being the richest in isoflavones. This is very high compared to the western diet, in which women would have an intake of somewhere between 2 and 5 mg of isoflavones a day. Translating this to therapeutic value, 40 mg isoflavone will be obtained by consuming 1.3 litres of soy milk, 35 grams of soy flour or 120 grams of tofu. The phytoestrogen levels in the blood and urine are up to twenty times greater in women from Asia, Central America or Mediterranean countries than in women from the west because a typical western diet has fewer legumes and vegetables rich in phytoestrogens than those in the Asian diet.

For this reason, the consumption of phytoestrogens as dietary supplements is on the rise in the west. Soy milk, soy-based breakfast cereals and soy and linseed breads are just a few products that are popularly consumed by postmenopausal women. Commercially available dietary tablets, such as Promensil, a red clover-based product, Remifemin, a black cohosh extract, and PhytoLife Soy are also popular plant oestrogen products that are widely promoted by their companies to pharmacies, health food stores and supermarkets as dietary supplements for women unable or unwilling to take hormone replacement therapy.

Women should also be aware that taking excessive doses of phytoestrogens might not be acceptable. Eating too much soy, tofu and legumes for the phytoestrogen effect, for example, might not be very palatable and could lead to flatulence and weight gain.

The clinical evidence for the beneficial effects of phytoestrogens at menopause has been obtained from epidemiological studies. But these need to be interpreted with caution because of the potential for bias. The major clinical application for phytoestrogens appears to be as an alternative source of oestrogen to treat hot flushes in postmenopausal women.

Early studies examining the effects of dietary isoflavone supplementation on menopausal symptoms produced inconclusive results due to the large placebo effects and to the small number of women studied. In a recent study published by Albertazzi *et al.* in *Obstetrics and Gynecology* (1998), 104 postmenopausal women were given daily supplements of either 60 g of soy or a placebo for twelve weeks. Reduction in hot flushes by 45 per cent was seen in the group that received soy, compared to a 30 per cent decrease in hot flushes from the placebo group. Similarly, studies conducted in Melbourne by Alice Murkies and her colleagues and published in *Maturitas* (1995) show a significant decrease in postmenopausal hot flushes over twelve weeks of using soy flour and wheat. It appears that dietary supplementation with phytoestrogens does help alleviate some menopausal symptoms.

Although there is a convincing pool of evidence to support the claim that phytoestrogen in the diet alleviates the number and severity of hot flushes, given that reporting hot flushes is very subjective, the effect of phytoestrogens still remains to be clarified.

'I sought assistance from a Chinese herbalist for treatment and acupuncture. I haven't had a migraine since that treatment.'

LORETO DAVEY

Epidemiological studies have also stimulated interest in the role that diets high in phytoestrogens may play in the prevention of diseases, such as cardiovascular disease and osteoporosis, as an association has been identified between high phytoestrogen intake and low incidence of cardiovascular disease. According to a 1993 World Health Organization report, Japanese and Chinese women who consume high levels of phytoestrogens have the lowest rate of cardiovascular disease. Animal studies also show favourable lipid levels in monkeys fed on a high soy diet. There have been no long-term studies that show with certainty that diets high in phytoestrogens have a beneficial effect on cardiovascular and bone health in postmenopausal women.

Although there is considerable interest in the potential use of phytoestrogen supplements in the prevention of cardiovascular disease, human research studies so far do not support the hypothesis that isoflavonoid phytoestrogens might improve cholesterol levels or serum lipid levels in people with average serum cholesterol concentrations. A randomised, double-blind, placebo-controlled trial with forty-six healthy men and postmenopausal women conducted in Western Australia, for example, and published by Hodgson *et al.* in the *Journal of Nutrition* in 1998, shows no improvement in high-density lipoprotein (HDL) and low-density lipoprotein (LDL) cholesterols after eight weeks of red clover intervention. (HDL is the 'good', more protective type of cholesterol; LDL is the 'bad' cholesterol.) However, studies in hypercholesterolaemic patients show that soy protein improves lipid profile (Anderson *et al.* 1995).

Research conducted in Melbourne by Nestel *et al.* in 1997 and published in *Arteriosclerosis, Thrombosis and Vascular Biology* found arterial compliance, that is, increased elasticity of the arteries and their ability to respond appropriately to increased blood volume, improved by 26 per cent in twenty-one women taking 80 mg of isoflavones daily for up to ten weeks when compared to a placebo.

'I went to school with one of the pioneers in this field, Jean Hailes, and I had great admiration for the job she did. But it was a real uphill job at the time she began her work. Nobody was interested. Hot flushes were thought to be nothing more than a bar-room joke.'

NANCY MILLIS

There have been no long-term studies of phytoestrogen supplementation showing beneficial effects on bone mineral density. It has been shown that populations with a high intake of dietary isoflavones have a low prevalence of osteoporosis. But a number of genetic and environmental factors could contribute to this, such as high calcium intake from early childhood, high levels of physical activity and an absence of smoking.

Most of the experimental studies have been performed on animals. As reported by Marco Messina at the International Menopause Society in Japan in 1999, phytoestrogens can retard bone loss in rats whose ovaries have been removed, although no positive effect on bone has been seen in monkeys fed a high concentration of soy.

Studies of phytoestrogen *in vitro* indicate favourable effects because it may slow the development of artherosclerosic disease. Other animal and human studies are potentially indicating a protective effect of phytoestrogens against bone loss.

Women in Asian countries have a low rate of hip fracture. Based on the limited studies published, it is not clear whether typical isoflavone intake in Asia is sufficiently high to prevent fractures, or whether this is due to the shorter length of the hip bone in these women when compared to Caucasian women, or other factors such as exercise.

The effects of phytoestrogens on cancer are supported only by epidemiological data. Many *in vitro* studies have shown that phytoestrogens can prevent breast and prostate cancer. Rose *et al.* (1986) have shown that populations with high levels of dietary phytoestrogens, such as Japan, have lower levels of breast and prostate cancer when compared to western counterparts. This might be due to the fact that isoflavones have an antioxidant effect and can mop up free radicals. Free radicals are highly unstable and reactive molecules, caused by many factors, including stress and pollutants. They attempt to stabilise themselves by attaching to body cells where they can cause damage.

A study conducted in West Australia by Ingram *et al.* and published in the *Lancet* in 1997, found that women with breast cancer had significantly lower urinary isoflavone excretions than controls, suggesting that phytoestrogen could be important in preventing breast cancer.

Studies in animals and *in vitro* demonstrate a range of mechanisms by which phytoestrogens may inhibit the formation and growth of cancer. But many of these effects have been demonstrated only at very high isoflavone concentrations.

Although the potential health benefits of phytoestrogens are still at an exploratory stage, it is fair to conclude that dietary supplementation with isoflavone phytoestrogens alleviates menopausal symptoms in some women and should be considered as an alternative therapy to oestrogen in women who cannot or do not wish to use hormone replacement therapy. The other postulated health benefits are inconclusive and show no hard evidence.

A large number of women seek help for their menopausal symptoms from alternative therapists, as well as from traditional medical practitioners. Chinese herbs, which have been used for centuries in China to treat postmenopausal symptoms, have increased in popularity in the west in the last ten years. It has been suggested that Chinese herbs such as Qing huo, Nuo dao gen and Panax ginseng possess oestrogenic effects that are effective in alleviating menopausal symptoms. But preliminary results of a study presented at the Australian Menopause Society in 1999 (Chen *et al.*), assessing the effectiveness of a specific Chinese herbal medicine in treating menopausal symptoms in Australian postmenopausal women, have not found the Chinese formula to be better in reducing the frequency of hot flushes and night sweats than a placebo. In another randomised trial reported by Hirata *et al.*, 1997, Dong Quai or 'female ginseng', a herb used by Chinese women for generations to ease menopausal symptoms, has been shown to be ineffective for menopausal symptoms.

'I think women have been conned: they are now expected to hold three jobs and really don't have choices at all, especially if they've got a husband and children.'

JEANNE PRATT

It appears that Chinese traditional medicine may be used effectively in treating postmenopausal symptoms in selected women only and in combination with hormone replacement therapy. You should consult a doctor of Chinese medicine for individual diagnosis. But Chinese herbs, like many other alternative and conventional therapies, do not provide protection from cardiovascular diseases and osteoporosis.

Certain herbal teas are known to have some therapeutic value and are used by naturopaths to treat hot flushes and sleeplessness in menopausal women. These herbs can be used fresh or dried and be prepared as teas or tinctures. Red clover and ginseng teas are rich in phytoestrogens.

Chamomile tea is useful for nervous tension and insomnia. Green tea is rich in antioxidant, phenols, and is associated with reduced cardio-vascular disease, and possibly with a reduced breast cancer incidence.

Susan Love in her comprehensive *Hormone Book* (1997) claims she has found a pool of evidence that black cohosh, sage, St John's wort and motherworth contain oestrogenic substances that can help alleviate hot flushes, night sweats, lethargy and insomnia. It has been shown that Remifemin, an extract of black cohosh, is better than a placebo. More common tea preparations for treating insomnia are chamomile and red raspberry leaf. Evening primrose oil and wild yam cream have failed to show improvements to menopausal symptoms over a placebo.

Lately progesterone creams have been promoted as effective in eliminating hot flushes and night sweats as well as preventing and treating osteoporosis. So far there have been no well-designed clinical trials that substantiate these claims. Recent published data on the use of topical progesterone showed that it did not achieve therapeutically significant blood levels and had no effect on the endometrium. In other words, the progesterone creams may not protect women from an increased risk of endometrial cancer.

Most of the claims that progesterone creams help menopausal women are based on anecdotal reports. Studies in the use of creams containing wild yam and evening primrose oil have shown both to be ineffective for menopausal symptoms.

Menopause is a time when you need to consider boosting your dietary intake of specific nutrients such as vitamins, essential fatty acids and minerals.

Vitamins are naturally occurring organic molecules needed in very small amounts in the diet for normal metabolic reactions in the body. They are essential for normal growth and health. They help in the for-mation of blood cells, maintaining strong bones and normal function of the heart and nervous system. Most vitamins cannot be synthesised by the body, so they must be consumed in food. The body can store the fat-soluble vitamins – A, D and E for later use, but it can't store water-soluble vitamins such as B and C so they must be constantly supplied in the diet.

Although many women take vitamin supplements in order to cope with the pressure of menopausal changes and to relieve some of the symptoms, most of these vitamins can be obtained in the diet. No calories are found in vitamins. If you take megadoses of vitamins, your body will excrete some, although most will be stored and in this way may become toxic.

Over-cooking food or eating too much processed food can lead to low levels of vitamins in your diet. The absorption of many vitamins can be affected by alcohol consumption and the use of some antibiotics. An increased vitamin intake might be required during emotional and physical stress. The best way to ensure that your body has enough vitamins is to eat a balanced diet, reduce the intake of alcohol, caffeine and salt, don't smoke and drink plenty of water.

A group of vitamins (A, C and E), also known as antioxidants, have surfaced as significant in combating various diseases.

Our bodies naturally create free radicals, especially when we are stressed or exposed to sunlight. But in the course of modern life, we encounter many more free radicals in smoke, toxins, chemicals and other pollutants in the air and in our food. Formation of free radicals leads to oxidation, which in turn leads to cell breakdown and tissue decay, resulting in internal diseases. Free radicals attack the repair mechanisms in the body and the genetic material responsible for cell reproduction (known as DNA) causing damage to, or cancer in, the internal organs.

A small number of free radicals cause unstable chemical reactions, triggering a chain reaction that can produce thousands more free radicals. Free radicals cause damage to the skin by causing loss of elasticity, discolouration and wrinkles.

Although the body manufactures cells that 'mop up' the free radicals, we can increase the supply of these neutralisers by increasing the supply of the antioxidant vitamins. But there is not enough evidence to support the intake of large quantities of antioxidants. 'Too much of a good thing' can backfire, so caution needs to be exerted when dosing yourself with supplements.

Vitamin E is often referred to as 'menopausal vitamin' as this vitamin may have chemical activity similar to oestrogen. This powerful vitamin seems to alleviate hot flushes and vaginal dryness, reduce insomnia and (as an antioxidant) it reduces the risk of heart disease and breast cancer. It is thought that vitamin E is most effective on the skin, as it appears to slow down the effects of ageing.

Deficiency of this vitamin may result in muscular weakness, tiredness and poor circulation. The best sources for vitamin E are oils found in wheat germ, vegetables, nuts, and in eggs, cabbage and spinach. Overdosing on vitamin E can cause hypertension and disrupt normal blood-clotting.

Vitamin C occurs naturally in all fruits and green vegetables especially kiwifruit, citrus fruit, tomatoes and bean sprouts. It is important for collagen formation on the skin, for healthy teeth, bones and gums, to build resistance to infection and to help wounds heal. Increased demands for vitamin C occur during stress, infection and when you have a poor diet.

Deficiency of vitamin C results in fatigue, irritability and lower resistance to infection. Over-consumption of vitamin C may cause diarrhoea and palpitations. You should consult a qualified health-care practitioner if you need to take supplements of this vitamin.

Vitamin A is important for the growth and health of the skin, eyes and mucous membrane. The nutrient Beta-carotene found in fruit and vegetables is converted to vitamin A in the liver. Vitamin A is a protective antioxidant for heart disease, cancer and cataract. It is found in green- and yellow-coloured fruits, apricots, mangos, peaches, watermelon and berries and vegetables such as carrots, sweet potatoes, red peppers, pumpkin and spinach. Excessive use of this vitamin can be toxic as the body has the ability to store it.

Consumption of processed foods, excessive coffee intake and taking hormone replacement therapy can deplete vitamin A, so adjust your diet accordingly.

Vitamin D, which is formed in the body as a result of exposure to sunlight, is essential for bone strength because it helps the absorption of calcium. Ten minutes in the sun each day should give you enough vitamin D for healthy bones. In some countries in the winter there is no sun, so two cups of milk each day would be sufficient for adequate vitamin D. Women who are confined indoors and are rarely exposed to sunlight should rely on their diet to provide sufficient amounts of vitamin D or use supplements each day that contain between 400 and 600 international units.

You also should include foods that are rich in vitamin D in your diet such as eggs, oily fish (salmon and sardines with bones) and dairy products, such as cheese.

All the B vitamins – B1 (thiamin), B2 (riboflavin), B2 (niacin), B5 (pantothenic acid), B6 (pyridoxine) and B12 (cyanocobalium) – work together to help various enzymes to handle blood sugar and stabilise brain function. Vitamins B6 and B12 are more helpful during the menopause as there is some evidence to show that these vitamins are useful for the relief of fluid retention.

It is known that hormone replacement therapy may lead to the depletion of Vitamin B6 and make you prone to depression. Vitamin B6 should not be taken in high doses as it can be toxic and cause nerve damage.

Vitamin B6 and B12 are found in fish, meat, and poultry; cereals and oats are a rich source of vitamin B2.

Essential fatty acids are important for cardiovascular health, calcium absorption, dryness of skin and vagina and hot flushes. Dietary sources of essential fatty acids include vegetable oils, especially flax seed oil, fish, dark green vegetables, alfalfa, kelp, liver, milk and egg yolk.

Minerals are as important as vitamins. They are inorganic compounds found naturally in the earth and, like vitamins, are needed in small quantities in order to maintain normal body health. The best sources of minerals are foods.

Menopause can affect the major building block of a woman's bones, which is calcium. The lack of the hormone oestrogen during menopause results in a significant loss of calcium, which can result in osteoporotic fractures in postmenopausal women.

As we age our body breaks down bone at a faster rate than it has the ability to replace it, which results in bones becoming more brittle.

Calcium is an important mineral for bone health. This mineral is essential to counter the increase in bone loss after menopause. Most of the body's calcium is found in our bones, and this makes up the bone mass.

In women, oestrogen helps calcium to be more effectively absorbed by the body. At about the age of forty, our bones start to lose calcium. After that age, women may lose up to 1 per cent of bone mass every year. As the oestrogen levels start to decrease at the onset of menopause, more calcium is lost from the bones – 2 to 3 per cent of bone mass each year. About 20 per cent of bone mass is lost in the first ten years after menopause, and this continues to decline at a slower rate as women get older.

Bone loss after menopause is the main reason that women, in particular, are at risk of osteoporosis. Statistics show that one in four Australian women will develop osteoporosis after the age of fifty. How much you lose calcium and the impact it has on your bones depends on genetic factors as well as how much calcium-rich food and drink you have consumed and how much exercise you have done in the first half of your life.

> 'Menopause is unavoidable as it is part of our natural physiology. What is important I believe is how we handle this phase of our lives. I sought the best advice available.'
>
> LORETO DAVEY

You can reduce the risk of bone loss by consuming foods that are rich in calcium. Dairy foods are best because they are especially high in calcium. Calcium-rich foods include milk, calcium-enriched soymilk, yogurt, cheese, ice cream, green vegetables such as beans, spinach silverbeet and cabbage, almonds, brazilnuts, hazelnuts and fish, such as sardines (especially with bones), salmon and flathead. Red meat and poultry are poor sources of calcium.

Calcium from dairy foods is more easily absorbed by the body than from nuts and vegetables. To avoid the fat content, skim milk or low-fat dairy foods should be consumed.

During digestion, calcium is absorbed from food. Vitamin D regulates the absorption of calcium. Lactose found in the milk also enhances calcium uptake by the body.

Women should refrain from smoking and from drinking too much coffee or tea. They should reduce their intake of salt, alcohol and foods rich in proteins, as these also increase the loss of calcium from bones and interfere with the body's ability to absorb calcium.

The amount of calcium you need each day depends on your age. The recommended dietary allowance for women between the ages of nineteen and fifty-four is about 800 to 1,000 mg a day. Postmenopausal women need between 1,300 and 1,500 mg a day or slightly lower if they are on hormone replacement therapy. The intake of calcium should be spread evenly over the day as the body can absorb about 500 mg at a time. Approximately two cups of milk and one cup of yogurt will give you the recommended daily allowance of calcium.

It is best to obtain calcium from food, but if you can't meet your daily dietary requirements you can take calcium supplements in a form of calcium citrate, calcium carbonate or calcium gluconate. Talk to your doctor or pharmacist about the best calcium supplement for you.

'I haven't met a woman anywhere who has mentioned her "empty womb" when discussing menopause. I think that we are all absolutely delighted that we won't be having any more children.'

ITA BUTTROSE

Zinc is needed for hormone and brain function and building new tissues. Good sources are found in beef, liver, pork, seafood, whole grain cereals and peanuts. A deficiency of this mineral can lead to metabolic problems.

Iron is the mineral that helps in oxygen transport in your body and plays a great role in the blood production. Iron-rich foods should be incorporated in your diet. They are present in a variety of foods, such as red meats, liver, egg yolks, legumes, dried fruits and green vegetables.

Iron deficiency is more common among women than men. The symptoms are weakness, shortness of breath and poor appetite. Excessive menstrual bleeding may cause iron deficiency.

Other beneficial minerals include potassium, magnesium, iodine and selenium. Fortunately many of the foods mentioned here contain these minerals.

Overconsumption of vitamins and minerals can have adverse effects on the body; they can even be toxic. It is a lot more difficult to megadose on vitamins from foods than from supplements. But no matter what quantities of vitamins you consume, you won't reap all the benefits unless you live healthily.

In a later chapter, we discuss the benefits of physical exercise. That is only half of the health picture. The other half, the mental picture, is just as important. By this we mean taking time for relaxation, spending time doing things with friends, relatives and family. Learn to control stress: being stressed can make even the simplest situation difficult to deal with. Relaxation techniques can help reduce the effects of stress in our daily lives.

But controlling stress is a decision you must make. Things are as good or bad as we perceive them. Try not to worry. It will not solve the problem. Emotional control is a skill that can be acquired, and it can add years to your life.

It is important to identify the signs of stress. They can be of a physical nature, such as restlessness, heart palpitations, headaches and feeling shaky, or mental, such as not being able to concentrate, constantly worrying about trivial matters, or feeling anxious all the time, or a combination of them all.

Relaxation skills, such as deep breathing and muscle relaxation, can be easily acquired. There are lots of books written on relaxation but here is a simple technique.

Get comfortable, then relax your muscles in your body by tensing and then relaxing them, beginning from the fingers of your hands and working up through your body till your body feels light and relaxed. Close your eyes and concentrate on your breathing. Imagine peaceful and relaxing scenes. See yourself there, part of the scene, happy and relaxed. Stay in that position for fifteen to twenty minutes and you will really feel the difference. Then gently bring movement to your hands, feet and whole body to come out of this relaxed state.

This relaxation regime should be practised daily. A good way to relieve stress is to exercise three to four times a week for approximately thirty to forty minutes. Exercise is beneficial for the body but also great for your soul.

Some of the more readily practised alternative therapies are massage, acupuncture, homeopathy, naturopathy and reflexology.

Massage relieves tension, stimulates circulation and relaxes you. A great treat you can give yourself. The other therapies mentioned are thought to stimulate the body's vital energy. If you wish to pursue these complementary therapies, make sure the person you see is qualified, knowledgeable and experienced. The treatment of menopausal symptoms may involve a combination of two or three formulae and may vary from one woman to another.

'I don't want to muck around with nature unless I have to.
I believe I can control my mood swings by being aware
and treating this naturally.'

TONIA TODMAN

It is important to establish good sleeping patterns and a regular sleep routine so that you get an adequate amount of sleep. For good sleep make sure you have a firm, supportive mattress, get plenty of exercise, have a good balanced diet and avoid caffeine and alcohol intake at night.

A positive attitude is important at any time of life, but especially so around menopause, as it can overcome some of the psychological problems that arise during that time. Recognise the value of the skills and experience that you bring to your family, life and job. Discover new challenges or interests that will help you feel better. Take time to do something you really like. Educate yourself as much as possible about menopause and learn how to cope with the changes your body is going through. Improve the quality of your life by implementing some of the changes we have discussed in this book. It is your turn to make these choices and enjoy life.

It is important to share the difficulties you are experiencing while going through menopause, with your husband or partner, children, family or friends. Explain how you feel and seek their support, understanding and encouragement. Communication is vital at this stage of your life.

By incorporating a well-balanced diet that is high in fruit, vegetables, cereals and legumes into your life, undertaking a regular exercise program and using relaxation techniques in your daily activities you can celebrate menopause and enjoy the years ahead.

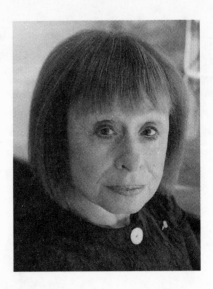

Jeanne Pratt, AO, was born in Lowicz, Poland, but came to Australia as a baby. As a young woman, she worked as a journalist, then became publisher of the *Women's Weekly* and reporter for the *Daily Telegraph* and the GTV-9 program *No Man's Land*. After her marriage to Richard Pratt, she gradually acquired her reputation as a woman committed to community service, the arts and philanthropic endeavour. She is director of the philanthropic arm of the family business, the Pratt Foundation, and is patron to numerous community and institutional enterprises. She is Chair of The Production Company, a non-profit theatrical company established in 1999 to promote and showcase new and established theatre talent and to stimulate the theatre industry. When she and her husband became the owners of the National Trust classified property, Raheen, she took the lead in its meticulous restoration and imaginative extension. Her 'open house' hospitality at Raheen has become legendary in Melbourne. She has also found time to be a successful wife, mother and grandmother.

Jeanne Pratt

I had a hysterectomy when I was about forty-six, and my doctor recommended that I start hormone replacement therapy. He explained that there was no such thing as a Fountain of Youth, but hormone replacement therapy was the next best thing. I must say, I haven't missed a beat.

Even though I am sixty-five years old, I don't think anybody ever picks me for that age. Sometimes I think I'm ageless. My only problem is that I developed high blood pressure about two years ago, but I had no symptoms of that either, and it's controlled by tablets. The only thing I can say is that I'm probably already too old to die young.

I've had no symptoms of menopause whatsoever. I'm very rarely sick; in fact, I don't get sick, I haven't got time.

I come from a generation in which you got up in the morning and did whatever you had to do, and if you and the task finished at night that was great and you didn't sit about asking yourself, Am I happy? I'm too busy to do that.

I was lucky that I was born with a comparatively sunny disposition, in the sense that I don't get mood swings, I'm pretty even. The only time I get upset is if there is something genuine to get upset about. Other than that I don't walk about asking myself if I'm happy; it's something I've never worried about.

I've never had a problem with lack of energy or loss of libido and I was never worried about moving into my unreproductive years.

I do not remember ever discussing my menopause with others, because everyone I knew was always on hormone replacement therapy and they didn't have any problems. The only one who did was actually my hairdresser who was about ten years younger than me, and she went through a difficult period. She lost her memory and she became quite distressed. But as soon as she went on hormone replacement therapy she was fine.

When you're really busy and focused on what you're doing, you don't have time to sit around worrying about how you feel.

During my menopause life went on as normal. I've done things at different ages from other people. I was on television at forty, for example – a new career at forty on television. And now, at the age of sixty-five, I've just started an entire theatrical company. There are only three of us running it: the manager, my secretary and me. Some bureaucracies would hire a couple of hundred people to do what the three of us do, so I don't think you could say I'm lacking in energy.

I've never given a thought to my appearance. I've never been preoccupied with my looks and I've always tried to develop my personality rather then worry about how I look. I don't think your personality ages necessarily, and I've always mixed with people of all different age groups.

I think it's a shame if someone has been a great beauty and has relied on this. It makes life very easy while they still have their looks. I don't intend to look any different from the way I do now for the rest of my life. If you look at Sheila Scotter, for instance – I mean she's eighty, very good looking and extremely glamorous. I always remember Scott Fitzgerald saying that, although his daughter was very beautiful, he advised her to play her cards as if she was a plain girl.

If you develop other aspects of yourself, ageing doesn't matter. I don't understand why it's such a big deal looking young. I like to look good for myself.

I think if you become physically unwell, people talk about the arrogance of good health. When you're healthy you just take it for granted, but I think you would very quickly feel otherwise if you became ill. So I'm not arrogant about that and I honestly don't think about my health very much. I've always got jobs to do. And I love doing crosswords and playing Scrabble, and I adore reading.

My husband and I start our day at about 4.30, because that's the time he wakes up, and we finish our day about 2.30. If we have to go out at night, I come home and go to bed, and I'll sleep for a couple of hours then, because I don't get much sleep through the night. Then I get up and go out. We are always in bed by 10.30 every night because we leave wherever we are at ten, no matter where – people are used to us and so they know that's what we do. We have a different way of life from most people.

It's extremely important, as an older woman, to have power and money, because if you don't have power and you don't have money you do get pushed into a corner. Our society devalues women in a way it doesn't men. And by power I don't mean you've got to be Prime Minister, but you must have control over something in your life so that you're not seen as an object or a victim. That's just my observation. It's nothing I have felt personally because I have not been in that situation, but I observe this, and I say to all women that it's very important they get some power in their life – and some money.

As women get older, they live very much in the present. I think when you're young, you always live in the future, but when you're old you tend to live very much in the present. I know a lot of older people who live in the past. I suppose I am an old person, although I've never thought of myself in that way. There's a life to be lived, but I don't live in the future and I don't live in the past. I live very much in the present.

I don't have a five-year plan, but perhaps I never did anyway. My husband has often said to me, 'What is your plan for blah, blah, blah?' But I don't have plans at all. I get asked to do a lot of things, so I've never had to ever look around for what am I going to do next. I think that would be a terrible thing to wake up in the morning and think, I've got a whole day, and what will I do? If it's a problem for other women, it's never been my problem. And I'm lucky like that.

I've been given a terribly interesting job offer, which I'm going to have a look at. The mayor of Jerusalem was here a few months ago and he's asked me would I restore and build a centre for performing arts in Jerusalem. It's an old leper hospital and they want to use it as a showcase for their high-tech industry. It's restoring the old building and putting up a wonderful new one.

The trouble is that I get so many interesting offers I'm a bit of a bridesmaid dancing at too many weddings.

I never did much exercise until I had problems with my blood pressure.

When my doctor examined me he said, 'Do you do any exercise?'

And I said, 'The only exercise I do is looking around for the nearest couch to sit down on.'

He said, 'That's no good. Now, let me take your blood pressure.'

My blood pressure was alarming, off the map, it was really, really high and I had no symptoms whatsoever. He put me on medication and, every Friday, I go for a walk with four friends, play croquet or do exercises, and then we have a cup of tea or coffee.

Would you really call this exercise? I've always lived on stairs. I run up and down about a hundred times a day so really that is my exercise.

The same with my eating. I really don't have a regime either.

In the morning I have a slice of toast with some cottage cheese and a cup of tea. I have a cellulite tablet and then I have a Renitec tablet, then I take vitamin B – one in a capsule – for calcium, and half a Disprin. That's what I take every day.

I tend not to eat much. I might have a cup of tea or coffee, but I don't ever eat cake, or very rarely, and only if I've got someone here will I eat before lunch. I usually have lunch at 12.30, and I usually have a vegetarian pizza or pasta. Occasionally I'll have a meat dish, but that's my main meal.

I might have a handful of nuts or something at 4.30, then at night time there's a chef who leaves food, and we tend to go up and down the stairs and just have a mouthful as we walk past. But we don't sit down and have meals every night. The only time we have meals at night is if we have visitors or if we go out. If they give you three courses, I might have a mouthful of every course. Somehow I don't think of it as a diet. It is just something that I do. If I'm starving I'll have a chocolate or whatever I want. My stomach I think must have shrunk over the years.

When my mother was about forty, she weighed about eleven stone. She had a massive heart attack at fifty and everyone in her family died before they reached fifty. She had only a very small part of her heart working at the end, and she had osteoporosis badly. I seem to have none of that and I really attribute that to being on hormone replacement therapy.

I usually have a mammogram once every two years, even though there's no cancer in my family, but I think it's well worth the trouble.

I've just put myself on a particular regime for taking hormone replacement therapy, and it may be totally wrong. I'm on it for four weeks and I go off it for one week – I've still got my ovaries – so I've decided to keep going with it, probably until I die. I've been lucky.

Nowadays I think people are so driven by what they do, rather than who they are, that they feel inadequate. A hundred years ago people used to ask about your family and no one was interested in what you did or how rich you were. Nowadays they ask you what do you do, and I get really cross when people say, 'I'm just a housewife.' I think it's more accurate to say, 'I am a general manager.' I think women have been conned: they are now expected to hold three jobs and really don't have choices at all, especially if they've got a husband and children. I've yet to see a husband who does anything around the home.

Chapter Six
Diabetes

What is diabetes? Type 1 and type 2. How to manage diabetes. What the onset of menopause means for women with diabetes. Cholesterol and the risk of cardiovascular disease. The effect of hormone replacement therapy on women with diabetes: the recent clinical studies, the advantages and potential risks.

Diabetes is an increasing concern in Australian society. According to the latest report released by the International Diabetes Institute in Melbourne, 940 000 Australians aged twenty-five and over have type 2 diabetes, with just as many undiagnosed cases. It is postulated that 1.2 million Australians will be affected by the year 2010.

Diabetes mellitus is a condition whereby the body cannot sufficiently convert ingested food into usable energy which results in disturbance in the blood sugar balance, causing high blood glucose, hyperglycemia. Fasting plasma glucose levels greater than 7 mmol/L are indicative of diabetes mellitus.

Everyone has sugar in their blood. Glucose comes from the carbohydrate foods we eat such as sugars and starches. When we consume carbohydrate-rich foods, they are broken down to simple sugar molecules, which in turn are absorbed into the blood and carried into the body's cells via the blood. Some glucose is used immediately as energy, while some of it is stored in the liver for subsequent slow release. Sugar is transported from the blood and into the body's cells by a hormone known as insulin, which is produced by a gland known as the pancreas.

After we have consumed food containing carbohydrate, the pancreas begins to release insulin into the blood circulation. The function of insulin is to maintain blood sugar levels within the normal range by helping the sugar to enter the body's cells.

Type 1 diabetes is also known as insulin-dependent diabetes mellitus (IDDM) or juvenile onset diabetes. It occurs when the pancreas stops producing insulin. This type of diabetes is seen in children and young adults, before the age of fifteen, and accounts for approximately 15 per cent of all diabetes. IDDM is an auto-immune disease which may be triggered by a virus or other environmental factors, and it cannot be prevented.

An auto-immune disease is one when the body's own immune system incorrectly identifies the pancreatic cells that produce insulin as 'foreign' and starts attacking and destroying them. Under these conditions the pancreas cannot produce sufficient insulin for the body's needs and diabetes occurs. Treatment of this form of diabetes includes working out a healthy diet plan, getting regular exercise and using regular injections of insulin.

Type 2 diabetes is known as non insulin-dependent diabetes mellitus (NIDDM) or mature onset diabetes. It occurs when the pancreas is unable to make sufficient amounts of insulin and the body cannot use the insulin effectively. Type 2 diabetes is more common in Australia and accounts for approximately 85 per cent of all diabetes. Type 2 diabetes usually appears after the age of thirty in adults who might be overweight and inactive or in women who have developed diabetes during pregnancy (gestational diabetes). The exact cause is unknown, but family history, and lifestyle factors such as overeating and obesity, have both been linked with its incidence increasing with age.

The symptoms of type 2 diabetes, such as frequent passing of urine, excessive thirst and weight loss, develop slowly and may go unnoticed for a long time, especially in the early years before diabetes is diagnosed.

This is usually combined with high glucose and insulin levels, high blood pressure and high lipid levels.

Up to half of all people with type 2 diabetes are not aware of it as in the early stages of the disease there are often no symptoms, and it is likely that an even larger number of people go undiagnosed. At the same time, a third of all people who are newly diagnosed with diabetes have evidence of vascular complications, which may have been preventable with early diagnosis and treatment.

Treatment of this form of diabetes includes developing a healthy diet and getting regular exercise. Weight reduction is of key importance if the person is overweight. It is also important to reduce fat intake and increase consumption of food with a low glycemic index. If the blood sugars remain high, however, treatment in the form of tablets may be required.

Poorly controlled diabetes may lead to a variety of conditions associated with the small blood vessels, known as microvascular diseases, which can affect the eyes (retinopathy) and kidneys (nephropathy). In addition, complications of the large blood vessels are common and may lead to cardiovascular disease, which is the leading cause of death among those with type 2 diabetes.

Irrespective of what type of diabetes you have, it is important to keep fasting blood sugar levels within the normal range (between 4 and 7 mmol/L) to prevent abnormal swings in blood sugar and to minimise the risks of long-term complications in the eyes, kidneys, nerves or blood circulation.

If you have diabetes it is very important to look after yourself properly and to manage the diabetes correctly. Improper care can cause damage to the blood vessels, which might lead to blindness, kidney failure, stroke or problems with your feet.

Understanding the principles of diabetes and your own treatment plan is imperative if you are to control and manage your diabetes. By taking good care of diabetes, it is possible to lead a long, healthy and active life.

To do this you need to take regular measurements of your blood glucose levels, and keep your weight under control by maintaining a structured diet and exercise program. You should exercise for at least thirty to forty minutes six days each week. Other changes should include stopping smoking, reducing high lipid levels (drug therapy may be needed) and controlling hypertension.

Recent trials in diabetic patients with hypertension indicate that rigorous control is important in reducing mortality from cardiovascular diseases.

At the 10th annual North American Menopause Society in 1999, Dr Tuck presented some alarming figures: in the US an estimated 14 per cent of white women, 23 per cent of black women, and 37 per cent of Hispanic women aged sixty have type 2 diabetes.

'Our periods might be necessary, but they certainly are a nuisance and, as far as I'm concerned, stopping them for good is a damn good idea.'

NANCY MILLIS

An alteration in glucose metabolism, often present with type 2 diabetes, may be associated with diminishing oestrogen levels in menopause. Oestrogen decline is also associated with an increased incidence of cardiovascular disease. Age and menopause significantly add to this vascular risk profile. As a result, cardiovascular disease in postmenopausal women with type 2 diabetes is very serious.

The high incidence of cardiovascular disease in postmenopausal women is exacerbated with type 2 diabetes. Results published about fifteen years ago by Feingold and Siperstein show that cardiovascular disease is the leading cause of death among people with type 2 diabetes, occurring earlier and more commonly than in people without diabetes. These authors go further and say that diabetic women have between three and seven times higher the relative risks for dying from cardiovascular disease than non-diabetic women.

As we see in other chapters, menopause is associated with changes in the lipid profile as well as an increase in blood pressure in non-diabetic women, two unfavourable factors for cardiovascular diseases.

High blood pressure, or hypertension, commonly occurs in diabetics, and represents an important health problem. Postmenopausal women with diabetes and hypertension are at increased risk of developing coronary heart disease and stroke compared to diabetics with normal blood pressure.

Diabetes can engender long-term vascular complications causing damage to the small blood vessels in the eyes, the kidneys and the feet, leading in turn to blindness, renal failure, gangrene and amputation. Health care in cases of diabetes is therefore very often preoccupied with the effects of these complications.

Treatment of insulin resistance and hyperglycemia can prevent or delay the vascular complications of diabetes, which are more prevalent and severe in women.

Diabetes is also associated with abnormal blood lipid profiles such as cholesterol. It is well documented that diabetic menopausal patients show decreased levels in the beneficial cholesterol (HDLc) and increased levels in the harmful cholesterol (LDLc). When the two cardiovascular factors, high blood pressure and an abnormal lipid profile, are combined, it is clear that the onset of the menopause in diabetic women could impose a great risk of cardiovascular disease.

Some women suffer from depression associated with diabetes and menopause. Such feelings need to be shared with your doctor and symptoms treated accordingly. Women at menopause, especially those with a history suggesting impaired insulin function, need to be monitored regularly, including for their diet and exercise. On an individual basis, diabetic women might need to receive specific treatment for menopause in the form of hormone replacement therapy, as well treatment for hypertension, hyperglycemia, hyperlipidemia and depression.

Postmenopausal women commonly use hormone replacement therapy to alleviate acute and chronic symptoms of the menopause. Postmenopausal women who take hormone replacement therapy are protected from cardiovascular diseases due to improved lipid levels. Hormone replacement therapy increases beneficial lipid profile (HDL) and reduces harmful lipid circulation (LDL) thus reducing the likelihood of atherosclerotic formation. Observational research studies published by Stampfer and Colditz in 1991 show that oestrogen replacement therapy has been associated with a 44 per cent decrease in the risk of cardiovascular diseases.

Although hormone replacement therapy, in its tablet form, is effective in reducing risk factors associated with cardiovascular disease, it has adverse effects on glucose metabolism, a condition that is already disturbed in diabetic women.

> 'Growing old is a pain in the butt. We all have to pretend we don't mind, but what a lie that is. Unless you go to a plastic surgeon and have a nip and tuck or whatever they all get done, what else can you do about it?'
>
> ITA BUTTROSE

Until recently, however, there have been no published studies on the effects of hormone replacement therapy in diabetic women. Longitudinal studies reported by Manson *et al.* in 1992 show that the use of hormonal replacement therapy does not increase the risk of developing diabetes later in life.

In the past four years, results from several interventional trials have been published, including those by Andersson *et al.*, Brussaard *et al.*, and Friday, which assessed hormone replacement therapy in women with non insulin-dependent diabetes. The studies have shown that treatment with oral oestrogen only, for up to three months, has several potential benefits for women with this kind of diabetes. It lowers blood glucose levels without increasing insulin levels and improves the lipid profile, with increased levels of beneficial lipids and decreased levels of harmful lipids, and no increase in triglycerides. Overall these studies showed an improvement in glucose metabolism.

As a result, hormone replacement therapy may occupy a place in the primary prevention of cardiovascular disease in diabetic postmenopausal women. Most of the studies conducted so far have been for short periods of time and have measured parameters assessing cardiovascular risks. We still do not know whether these potential beneficial cardiovascular effects will translate into actual protection against cardiovascular events.

Women with an intact uterus must also take progesterone to prevent uterine cancer. Hardly any studies have been done on the effects of combined hormone replacement therapy (oestrogen and progesterone) in postmenopausal diabetic women, although it is thought that the type of progesterone used, synthetic or natural, may influence the end results.

'I never really thought that the onset of menopause was a sign that I was growing old. It was simply something that you lived through while you got on with the real job.'

JOAN KIRNER

Our own studies underway at Victoria University will examine the effects of a new hypoglycemic treatment alone or in combination with a hormone replacement regimen in reducing cardiovascular risk factors, preventing osteoporosis and maintaining normal glucose metabolism in postmenopausal women with type 2 diabetes.

From the studies discussed above, it appears that, in addition to the beneficial cardiovascular effects, homone replacement therapy improves glucose metabolism and insulin sensitivity in diabetic women, which is usually of great concern for clinicians when treating diabetic patients.

The potential risks of hormone replacement therapy for diabetic women include worsening of triglycerides, already known to be an independent cardiac risk factor for women with diabetes, as well as some increased risk of developing deep venous thrombosis and pulmonary embolism.

In diabetic women, careful choice of the type and dose of hormone replacement therapy is required as not all regimens produce favourable results. It is not fully known what effects combined hormone replacement will have on women with diabetes, although some types of progesterone are known to worsen insulin resistance. It appears that synthetic progestins such as medroxyprogesterone acetate (MPA) and levonorgestrel increase insulin resistance and decrease glucose tolerance. In addition synthetic progestins appear to be more harmful in decreasing the beneficial cholesterol levels, thus offering less protection against cardiovascular diseases than the natural progesterones such as norethisterone acetate (NETA), dydrogesterone or micronised progesterone in oestrogen/progestin regime.

Few studies have evaluated the effects of oestrogen alone or oestrogen with progestins in diabetic women. There are some studies that have investigated glucose and insulin metabolism in non-diabetic postmenopausal women, such as the PEPI trial, showing that oestrogen in low doses has a favourable effect on glucose and insulin metabolism.

Overall, it would appear that hormone replacement may have a number of benefits for women with type 2 diabetes. But given the potential risks and the fact that there have been no long-term clinical trials to evaluate its effects, clinicians need to exercise great care when prescribing hormone replacement therapy for women with type 2 diabetes.

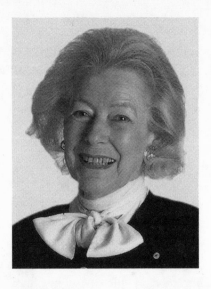

Sheila Scotter, AM, started her fashion career as a model and ended it as editor-in-chief of *Vogue* in Australia. She was also the founding editor of *Vogue Living* magazine. Born in India and educated in England, in 1949 she was brought to Australia by Myer Emporium to buy imported clothes for and run their Model Salon in Melbourne. Georges of Collins Street then appointed her their high fashion director. In 1956 she started the marketing division Everglaze and Banlon for textile company Joseph Bancroft & Sons of the US, who later moved her to the top job in Paris where she lived for four and a half years. In 1961 Conde Nast Publications brought her back to Sydney to edit *Vogue*. She was editor for over nine years and was awarded an MBE for services to journalism and commerce. Later, Sheila wrote regularly for the *Australian Women's Weekly*, the *Age* and *Home Beautiful magazine*. Random House published her autobiography, *Snaps, Secrets and Stories of My Life*. One of Australia's best-known social figures and fundraisers, Sheila was made an AM in the Order of Australia for services to the arts in 1972.

Sheila Scotter

I started the 'curse', which was what we called menstruation in
England, when I was about sixteen. Although I had the odd pains that
you usually got for the first two days of your period, I never had
headaches, or anything like that, and I never got moody. I think I was
around forty-eight when I reached menopause. And just as it had been
with my periods, it never really caused me any trouble at all.

My mother told me not to worry about anything during
menopause. She said that a lot of women go on about it, but in reality
it's very little trouble. Her advice must have worked. I suppose I have
her strong genes to thank for that.

I wasn't too upset to come to the end of my cycle. I didn't intend
to have any children. I'd been married twice already, and there were no
plans to have a family. I don't mind not having any children of my
own. All of my love goes to other people's children.

In our family we never talked about women's things, like
menstruation and, of course, you never discussed anything like that
with your father, but you would compare things with the odd
girlfriend.

Lots of my girlfriends had problems. They would say things like,
'I can't go out this weekend, it's awful for me.' And they would have
a terrible build up and then trouble throughout their periods. But I

never had any of that, not at all. Then my periods began to ease off, and then take me by surprise when they returned. When you were much younger, you always cursed your period, especially when it affected your sporting activities.

It was pretty much the same with my menopause. I had no hot flushes or sweats, nothing. It seemed like everybody else I talked to had hot flushes, but I never got those.

I went to *Vogue* when I was about forty-two. I was editor-in-chief around the time I reached menopause. I can't remember exactly, but I think I was forty-eight when my periods stopped altogether. Like most women, I knew when my period was coming, I suppose every month, but I didn't really take that much notice of it.

I have always been very busy and full of energy. Maybe that's why I've never been concerned about growing old. But right now I'm eighty and I've started to think, Well, now I'm old, there's no question about it.

I've never disguised my age, after all, it's always been there. If anything, I have always boasted about it.

I've had an extraordinary life. Even though my family were all in England and I was out here, I've always had lots of friends. I never really had to think about my financial status because I was always moving up and on with my career.

I'm lucky enough to have never asked for a job. I've always been told to do one or had one offered to me. I've had some crazy offers. Like the time I was asked to come and run the marketing division for some big American company.

I said, 'But I don't know anything about marketing.'

And they said, 'Oh, yes you do.' And before I knew it, I had the job.

As far as healthy living goes, I walk a bit, but I try not to overdo it. I have always eaten properly, but I have a small appetite. I don't like big helpings. I always have regular good food and nothing that is too fattening. I've never craved pudding, or things like that. If I'm alone, like I was today for lunch, I make myself something quick, like a gorgeous pasta. I eat vegetables, salad, fruit, meat or some kinds of fish.

I always cook something. Sometimes I have a delicious piece of cheese with fresh bread and tomato, something like that. I always eat breakfast too. I have a boiled egg, a couple of pieces of toast and a cup of coffee.

I've never really done any exercise. I walk a bit, but I don't count that as a real exercise program. If I'm going up and down stairs, then that's something a bit extra.

I've never had any regular medical check-ups, although I did have a pap smear once. As for mammograms, I honestly don't believe in them. Sometimes they don't pick up abnormalities or anything. I did have a mammogram when the caravan came round once. My breast surgeon, asked me why I had never had one before and I told him that I couldn't be bothered. I've known so many women who have had problems, but nothing showed up in the initial screening.

I first realised that I had some kind of problem when I started losing weight, going back to almost the weight I was when I was a model. At the time I must have been slightly overweight for my height. I was on this medication for a bit and I said to my doctor, 'Look, I'm losing weight.' I don't have any scales at home, but I judge my weight by my figure – whether skirts or pants feel too tight or the belts are too loose. So my doctor weighed me and I had dropped to 59 kilos or something like that. I was usually about 68 kilos, but not fat. Then my bosoms got a bit smaller – they were always small anyway – and that's when I noticed the lump.

My general health has been amazing throughout my whole life, until the lump in my breast. It's only now that things are beginning to trouble me, which is annoying. I've had the wretched lump removed two and a half years ago. The operation was successful, and my check-ups have been all clear since then.

I think I must have inherited some very good genes. My parents were the same – they never had any illnesses at all. We certainly never had any bloody cancer in the family – until me. So many women seem to get breast cancer these days.

Now, I am in reasonable health and definitely plan to enjoy my older years.

Chapter Seven
The breast

The effects of hormones and other factors on the breasts. Causes of common breast symptoms (pain, lumps, nipple discharge) and some solutions and treatments. Why does breast cancer develop? How do doctors investigate a breast lump? The causes of breast cancer. How breast cancer is treated. Studies into the effectiveness of some treatments: Tamoxifen, Raloxifene, phytoestrogens, aromatase inhibitors. Studies into hormone replacement therapy in relation to breast cancer.

Many women experience breast symptoms during their forties or peri-menopausal years. These symptoms are usually related to fluctuating hormonal changes. Breast symptoms are very common in women throughout their child-bearing years. Many symptoms can be attributed to the effects of the ovarian hormones, oestrogen and progesterone, on the breast tissue. The production of these hormones varies throughout the menstrual cycle.

Oestrogen is the predominant hormone in the early (follicular) stage of the cycle and around ovulation. Progesterone has an action on breast tissue in the latter (luteal) stage of the cycle. Breast discomfort in the week before the period is commonly related to the hormones causing fluid retention in the breast tissue. Fluid retention occurs causing swollen, painful breasts. Other hormones such as the pituitary gland hormones, prolactin and oxytocin, also play a role in breast changes. Prolactin is a hormone that is produced by the pituitary gland – a small gland at the base of the brain. Prolactin helps in the production of milk in breast-feeding women.

Hormonal changes interact with other factors. Stress may increase your prolactin level and this, in turn, produces pain or discomfort in the breast.

In women who go to their doctor with symptoms related to the breast, 95 per cent of these are caused by benign breast conditions and about 5 per cent by breast cancer. Symptoms include breast pain (mastalgia), nipple discharge and breast lumps. Mastalgia is usually a result of hormonal changes or benign breast cysts, but occasionally breast discomfort can be related to breast cancer. Breast lumps are either caused by benign or malignant conditions.

Mastalgia is very common. About 60 per cent of women complain of breast pain at some stage during their child-bearing years. It is usually mild and related to the normal pre-menstrual hormonal changes acting on the breast tissue. Mastalgia can also occur due to an infection in the breast. Breast infections commonly occur in breast-feeding women. Infections in the breast are usually treated with antibiotics.

Generalised lumpy, or nodular, breasts are very common. Breasts tend to be lumpier before menstruation, and breast discomfort – either swelling or pain – generally abates after a period.

Non-cyclical breast pain occurs in perimenopause and is often a result of the relative hormonal chaos common in women in their forties. The hormonal changes that cause erratic periods are reflected in the symptoms that come and go in the breast. It is not uncommon for women to experience markedly sore breasts during some cycles and few symptoms during others. Breast pain can be improved by reducing caffeine intake, which reduces fluid retention in breast tissue. A low-fat, high-fibre diet and a low alcohol intake (fewer than two alcoholic drinks each day) are recommended. Supplements such as evening primrose oil capsules (1,000 to 2,000 mg a day) and vitamin B6 (100 mg daily) may also be helpful.

If the breast pain is more severe and becomes chronic, other treatments used include anti-inflammatory drugs, progestogens (starting very early in the menstrual cycle), Danazol and, rarely, Bromocryptine and Tamoxifen. Tamoxifen acts as an anti-oestrogen drug on breast tissue by inhibiting or countering the effect of oestrogen on the breast. It is used commonly in women who have had breast cancer. More recently, it has been used in clinical trials for the prevention of breast cancer in women who may have a high risk of developing breast cancer. These include women who have a family history of breast cancer at an early age.

Nipple discharge is a less common symptom. A greenish fluid discharge from several ducts may be associated with a benign condition called mammary duct ectasia. When a single duct produces a bloody

'Each of the doctors I went to said, "Well, what are you working for? You don't need to work." At that stage I was Commissioner for Corporate Affairs, and then I was President of the Equal Opportunity Board. I'm sure they would never say that to a man.'

JAN WADE

discharge, the cause is usually a small tumour that grows in the duct called a papilloma, which requires surgical removal.

Breast lumps occur in women in three distinctive age groups. In women between twelve and thirty-five the lumps are usually fibroadenoma, which are benign, mobile solid lumps within the breast tissue; between thirty-five and fifty-five years breast lumps are usually breast cysts.

Breast cysts are very common in women in their forties and early fifties if they are still menstruating or if they are on hormone replacement therapy. Breast cysts will often be detected in mammograms as a rounded white lump. Ultrasound examination will help determine whether the lump is solid or cystic. Ultrasounds can be safely used in pregnant and young women.

Breast lumps due to cancer can occur at any age but are a more common cause of a lump in older women. Breast cancer may appear as a firm to hard lump in the breast. Sometimes there will just be a firm thickened area that feels different from the other breast tissue. Any woman with a new lump appearing in breast tissue must have it checked by a doctor.

Regular breast self-examination is important. Becoming familiar with the texture and normal changes that occur before and after periods will help you to detect abnormal changes in the breast. The best time for examining breasts is after a menstrual period, because breasts tend to be less lumpy or tender at this time. Self-examination once a month is ideal.

An annual examination by a doctor is important. In women who are forty or over, mammograms every two years are recommended if they have no risk factors for breast cancer. If there is a family history in immediate relatives – mother, sister, or daughter – then yearly mammograms are recommended.

Age is the strongest risk factor for developing breast cancer. When looked at as a whole group, women from nought to eighty have a one in twelve risk (8.3 per cent) of developing cancer. When broken into age categories, this risk increases with age. Women in their twenties have a comparatively small risk (0.05 per cent) which increases to 0.4 per cent for women in their thirties. One in every sixty-nine women in their forties (almost 1.5 per cent) are at risk of developing cancer, and women in their fifties and sixties have around a 2.7 per cent chance of developing the disease. The other strong risk factor is a family history of breast cancer.

Inherited breast cancer accounts for 5 to 10 per cent of breast cancers. Breast cancer is likely to be genetic if the cancer developed in the relative at under forty years of age, there was cancer in both breasts (bilateral cancer), other cancers were present, for example, ovarian cancer, or at least two immediate relatives have breast cancer.

The most commonly inherited breast cancers are BRCA 1 and BRCA 2, which are thought to account for 90 per cent of inherited breast cancer. In genetically inherited breast cancer, an abnormality or mutation is present in all the cells in the body at birth. Although the cells in the body, including the breast cells, carry an abnormal gene, five or six other mutations must occur in the breast cell before it becomes a cancerous cell. This is why some women develop cancer at an earlier age than other women. The development of cancer depends on when these other mutations take place. Not all women who have a genetically mutant cancer gene will develop breast cancer. A cancer will only develop if the other mutations occur.

The development of a breast cancer is an interplay between genes and age, diet, socio-economic status, toxins, way of life, radiation and hormones. The other factors mentioned play a role in provoking further mutations in the cells. Breast cancer that is not a result of genetically inherited breast cancer genes is caused by somatic mutations. Somatic mutations occur spontaneously in only one type of cell in the body.

'Young women seem to think about what they eat, what they do, all aspects of their lifestyle, whereas my generation was a bit inclined just to get on with it.'

BARBARA CHAMPION

If you have a lump in your breast that concerns you, it is important to go to your doctor for a thorough check or to ask for a referral to a breast specialist.

Most breast cancer is detected after symptoms occur rather than through screening. Breast-screening mammograms, however, have been shown to be very useful in the detection of breast cancer lumps that are too small to be felt by examination. Early detection of breast cancer, when the lump is small, reduces the likelihood that the cancer has spread to other areas of the body. The impact on survival of delays between onset of symptoms and the start of treatment is controversial, but there does seem to be a survival advantage if the cancer is treated as early as possible.

Investigation of a breast lump will often involve some or all of these procedures: clinical examination, mammography, ultrasound, fine-needle aspiration (FNA), core biopsy, open biopsy, lumpectomy or mastectomy, axillary lymph-node dissection, pathological staging and establishing a woman's oestrogen/progesterone receptor status.

Fine needle aspiration is when a sample of a few breast cancer cells is taken using a syringe with a fine needle attached.

With core biopsy, several samples are taken from the lump with a thicker needle.

Open biopsy is removal of the lumpy area through an incision in the breast. It requires an anaesthetic.

Lumpectomy is removal of the lump in the breast plus a small amount of tissue surrounding the lump that is clear of cancer.

Mastectomy is removal of all the breast tissue on the side that contains the cancer.

Axillary node dissection is removal of the lymph glands in the armpit, as the cancer may have spread to this area. If it has spread to the lymph glands then chemotherapy is usually given to kill the cancer cells.

Pathological staging determines whether the cancer has more or fewer malignant cells – called differentiation of the cells – and whether there has been spread outside the breast tissue.

Breast cancer is the third most common cancer in the world. It accounts for 9 per cent of all new cancers and 18 per cent of all female cancers. Over 50 per cent of breast cancer incidence (490 000 cases in 1996) occur in western societies, such as Australia.

The areas of high risk include Europe, North America and Australia. The lowest rates occur in Asia and Africa. There is an increasing incidence in most countries, including areas that had a low rate previously. At least part of this increase, however, is due to early detection of cases by screening with mammography.

In the United Kingdom, for example, the incidence approaches two for every thousand women each year, and the disease is the single most common cause of death among women aged between forty and fifty. It accounts for about a fifth of all deaths in this age group.

In Australia, the lifetime risk of developing breast cancer is one in twelve, and one in twenty-five women will die of breast cancer. There is a 70 per cent, five-year survival overall, but a 90 per cent, five-year survival if the cancer is small when detected. There are about 700 new cases diagnosed in Australia each year and 2,400 deaths. The age-related incidence is increasing by 1 to 2 per cent each year, and with an ageing population there is an increasing prevalence. The strongest risk factor for breast cancer is age.

Much of the information women have about their risk of developing breast cancer is not based on fact. In 1996, the National Breast Cancer Centre (NBCC) surveyed 3,000 healthy women in Australia about their knowledge, attitudes and self-reported behaviour about breast cancer. The survey asked about risk factors for breast cancer, and only 5 per cent of women nominated age as a related cause. In response to the question, When is a women at greatest risk? most women (78 per cent) indicated that women in their forties and fifties were at greatest risk, while no more than 6 per cent suggested that women in their sixties had the highest risk of breast cancer.

These are the established and probable risk factors for breast cancer: geographical location, age at menarche (the time of your first period), age at menopause, age at first full pregnancy, family history, previous benign breast history, cancer in other breast, socio-economic group, poor diet, excess body weight, excessive alcohol consumption, use of hormone replacement therapy for more than five years, exposure to ionising radiation, taking exogenous hormones such as the contra-ceptive pill for more than four years, the use of Diethylstilbestrol during pregnancy and increasing age.

The rate of the increase in incidence of breast cancer slows at menopause. Women who have an early menarche, or late menopause, have an increased risk of developing breast cancer.

There is no definitive correlation between fat intake and breast cancer, although there appears to be a relationship between the incidence of breast cancer and the dietary intake of fat on a population basis. In other words, western societies that have a high dietary fat intake also have a high incidence of breast cancer. There is some indication from observational studies that there is a dose-response relationship between alcohol intake and breast cancer risk. The relative risk from the studies was in the range of 1.5 to 2.0. That is, there is about twice the risk if you drink more than two glasses of alcohol each day.

Evidence from randomised controlled trials, that is, trials in which women who had had mammograms were compared with those who hadn't, has shown that screening by mammography may reduce the mortality rate from breast cancer by 30 to 40 per cent. The age group that has the most benefit is over fifty years. Early trials did not show a benefit in the forty to fifty age group. In this age group, more frequent screening may be applicable. The usual interval is two years, with two views being obtained of each breast. Over 70 per cent of women in the population need to participate to significantly reduce mortality.

Ductal carcinoma in situ (DCIS) is apparently increasing in incidence. This increase, however, is related to mammographic screening. The natural history of DCIS is still poorly known. It is most commonly associated with micro-calcification, that is, minute deposits of calcium appear in the breast ducts, which are associated with the development of abnormal cells in the ducts. This micro-calcification is seen as little white dots on the mammogram.

Usually, these white dots are benign, or non-malignant. An experienced radiologist can often distinguish between benign calcification and calcification that is possibly due to a small cancer in the early stage of development. If there is any doubt, a biopsy of the breast tissue will usually be performed.

The micro-calcification may be localised or widespread throughout the breast tissue. From several studies it has been established that the proportion that progress to invasive cancer may be around 33 per cent. Widespread DCIS, which means DCIS throughout the breast tissue, is generally treated by mastectomy, and has a 98 per cent, five-year survival rate. At present, clinical trials are being conducted to determine the optimal treatment of screen-detected DCIS.

The treatment of breast cancer will depend on the size of the lump, its position, whether multifocal disease is present (that is, where cancer is occurring in several areas of the breast) and the stage of the cancer.

Favourable prognostic indicators include having a small tumour, the absence of lymph node involvement, positive oestrogen receptors and positive progesterone receptors. Positive oestrogen receptors are on cells that will respond or grow in response to oestrogen. Tamoxifen, an anticancer drug, can be used if oestrogen receptors are positive – thus stopping the growth of the cancer.

Many women with a diagnosis of breast cancer feel helpless or powerless. They are concerned about the threat to their life, the threat to their femininity, the impact on their family, whether the cancer will spread, and uncertainty about the future.

Most women will find it hard to understand the implications of a diagnosis of breast cancer. Many centres that treat women for breast cancer have a support service available. But seeking help from doctors and other health professionals is essential. Do not be afraid to ask questions or repeat them if you are not certain about the diagnosis and treatment plan. The more information you have, the more able you will be to take an active role in your future treatment.

Some areas of advancement in the prevention and treatment of breast cancer include genetic testing; adjuvant therapy, which is the use of chemotherapy or hormonal drugs, such as Tamoxifen, for node-negative women (women who don't have cancer detected in their glands); inhibition of ovarian function, for example, with Zoladex; new drugs that reduce the production of oestrogen, such as the aromatase enzyme inhibitors, for example Arimidex; and clinical trials with Tamoxifen in women at high risk for developing breast cancer. Tamoxifen has both oestrogenic and anti-oestrogenic effects. This drug is useful in preventing the recurrence of breast cancer in oestrogen receptor (ER) positive patients. Oestrogen receptor negative patients do not benefit. Tamoxifen treatment in ER positive patients results in a 47 per cent reduction in five-year recurrence and a 26 per cent reduction in mortality.

Tamoxifen has an effect on the endometrium and the ovaries. It increases the incidence of cysts on the ovaries and has been shown to cause a number of changes in the endometrium. These include hyperplasia (excessive increase in the thickness of the endometrium) and, uncommonly, endometrial cancer. An endometrial biopsy, which involves sampling the endometrium, and pelvic ultrasound is not necessary as a routine investigation in women on long-term Tamoxifen, as 66 per cent have a false positive rate with ultrasound. In other words, when a vaginal ultrasound is done on women who are on Tamoxifen, abnormalities appear to be present, but when a biopsy is done no abnormality is seen. Vaginal bleeding, however, is a symptom and in anyone taking Tamoxifen it needs to be discussed and investigated by a doctor.

International clinical trials are being conducted to evaluate the benefits of using Tamoxifen for the prevention of breast cancer in women at a high risk of developing breast cancer. One of the causes of concern is the increased risk of endometrial cancer in women on long-term Tamoxifen treatment. If Tamoxifen reduces the risk of developing breast cancer by 30 per cent (a rate that is similar to screening mammography), this will far outweigh the overall slight increase in the incidence of endometrial cancer.

'As far as I was concerned, menopause was a biological event. It was a bloody nuisance while it lasted, and when it was over I thought, Thank goodness for that. And that was it.'

NANCY MILLIS

Raloxifene is a new drug that belongs to a group of drugs called SERMS – selective oestrogen receptor modulators. Tamoxifen and clomiphene are related to Raloxifene. Raloxifene is a new medication for the treatment of osteoporosis with fracture.

During clinical studies with Raloxifene, it was noted that there was a reduced incidence of breast cancer in women on Raloxifene compared with those taking a placebo. In the United States, new research called the STAR study is underway as part of the National Surgical Adjuvant Breast and Bowel Study to compare Tamoxifen and Raloxifene. Raloxifene does not have the same effect on the endometrium as Tamoxifen. It has a positive (agonistic) effect on bone and blood lipids and a negative (antagonistic) effect on the breast and endometrium.

Epidemiological studies have shown that in nations where phytoestrogens, such as soya products and lentils, are consumed in the largest amounts the incidence and death rate from breast cancer is lowest. Phytoestrogens have a structure that is similar to oestrogen. The epidemiological studies do not prove that phytoestrogens have anti-cancer properties. Some pre-clinical trials, however, indicate some support for this concept. It may be that early life exposure to them is the critical factor for breast cancer prevention.

Women in countries with a diet high in phytoestrogens have fewer and longer menstrual cycles compared with western women. As a result the breast cell undergoes fewer mitoses (divisions). Clinical studies are underway to define the effect of phytoestrogens on breast cancer recurrence.

Aromatase inhibitors, that is, drugs that block the action of an enzyme called aromatase, have been used for the treatment of advanced postmenopausal breast cancer. The enzyme aromatase is involved in the pathway leading to the production of oestrogen. Several new aromatase inhibitors have been developed which are more effective and have less side effects than older drugs. These drugs are used if drugs such as Tamoxifen are no longer effective in patients with widespread cancer throughout the body.

Chemotherapy and drugs that block the production of oestrogen from the ovary, such as Zolodex, reduce death rates in breast cancer patients. An additional alternative later stage drug is Paclitaxel (Taxol).

The challenge with breast cancer is, firstly, to prevent its occurrence, particularly in high-risk women and, secondly, to detect it as early as possible and to use preventive strategies to reduce its recurrence.

There have been many individual studies and several meta-analyses (large studies that combine the results from several small studies) that have investigated the risk of developing breast cancer with the use of oestrogen or oestrogen/progestin regimes common in hormone replacement therapy. Many of these studies have shown no increase in the risk of breast cancer. But some have shown a small increase in the relative risk, usually with longer term use.

Unfortunately, there have been no long-term, randomised, placebo-controlled trials with sufficient numbers of women to give an answer to the question. It is clearly an important issue for many women. There are some large trials in progress, for example, the Women's Health Initiative (WHI) and the WISDOM study. The results of these studies, however, will not be available for several years. The WHI is a large, double-blind, randomised, controlled trial involving 275 000 women aged from fifty to seventy-nine. It has been specifically designed to resolve questions about the risks and benefits of hormone replacement therapy and will be completed in 2007.

In counselling women, we generally have to rely on the best available evidence and, ultimately, women should be able to make their own decision based on the knowledge that doctors are able to give them – information based on the present state of knowledge on the subject.

'I think our need to discuss and analyse menopause is a psychological pressure, a seed planted in our head. I think we need to avoid the pressure.'

JANNIE TAY

Two studies, published in the last few years, have been the focus of considerable discussion. One of these has been based on the Nurses' Health study, a long-term study of women who were regarded as 'healthy' at the beginning of the study in 1976.

This study reported a significant increase in the risk of breast cancer with long-term hormone replacement use, particularly its use for more than ten years, and particularly in the over sixty years age group. Adding progestins did not appear to decrease the risk. Some critics of the results of this study have pointed out that the HRT group received 14 per cent more mammograms than the non-users, and, as a result, asymptomatic cancers (cancers not causing symptoms) may have been detected. In their report, the investigators state that ductal carcinoma in situ (DCIS) diagnosed on the mammograms were not included in the results as cancers.

The second study, published in the *Lancet* in October 1998, reported on the accumulated epidemiological studies. Fifty-one studies performed over the last twenty-five years were used in the analysis (90 per cent of the worldwide studies). They re-analysed data on 52 705 women with breast cancer and 108 411 women without breast cancer.

The main analyses were on 53 865 postmenopausal women with a known age at menopause. 17 830 women (33 per cent) had used hormone replacement therapy at some time. The median age at first use was forty-eight years. Thirty-four per cent of the users had been on hormone replacement for five years or longer. The analyses took into account age at diagnosis, time since menopause, body-mass index, parity (number of children) and the age at which women had their first child.

Women who had used hormone replacement therapy for a period of one to four years had no increase in their risk of cancer. For women who used it for five years or longer, the relative risk was 1.35. This can be interpreted as a 35 per cent increase in the risk of breast cancer if oestrogen replacement therapy is taken by a woman starting at around the age of fifty – the normal age for natural menopause – and continuing until the age of fifty-five, or longer.

In North America, Europe and Australia the cumulative incidence of breast cancer between fifty and seventy in women who have never used hormone replacement therapy is forty-five per one thousand women. If it is used for five years forty-seven women in every thousand will develop breast cancer. If used for ten years, forty-nine in every thousand will develop breast cancer. That is, the risk of breast cancer increases with increasing duration of use. The study also found that this effect is reduced after stopping hormone replacement therapy and has largely disappeared after five years.

Despite the large numbers of women in this study, only 12 per cent of users had been exposed to progestins. The study had an insufficient number of women in this group to investigate individually oestrogen/progestin regimes and breast cancer risk.

Several epidemiological studies suggest that the risk for colorectal cancer may be diminished by the use of hormone replacement therapy.

The Nurses' Health study also evaluated the risk of bowel cancer in its large long-term study of women.

In the study, reported in the *Annals of Internal Medicine* in May 1998, the researchers found that use of hormone replacement therapy was associated with a decreased risk for bowel cancer. The relative risk was 0.65, that is, there appears to be a 35 per cent decrease in the risk of bowel cancer if hormone replacement therapy is taken for several years.

This effect disappeared five years after stopping hormone replacement therapy. Longer use did not provide any additional protection. The proportion of women who used hormone replacement therapy who were receiving a screening colonoscopy was 15.4 per cent. In the non-user group, the numbers were almost identical (15.8 per cent).

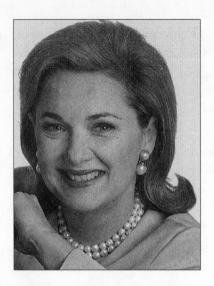

Tonia Todman was born in Queensland. Her
family moved to the island of Samarai, off the coast
of Papua New Guinea when she was two years old,
and she returned to Australia for her secondary
school education. After school she worked in various
office and administration jobs, before marrying at
twenty. After the birth of her children in the mid-
seventies she worked from home for *Vogue Patterns*,
sewing, teaching, running their fashion parades and
marketing new products. This continued for ten
years, merging with a burgeoning career in
journalism and photographic styling. She has been
involved with television for fourteen years,
including eight with *Healthy, Wealthy and Wise*. She
is now in demand as a public speaker. Her other
passions are gardens and cooking. After thirty years
in Sydney, she now lives in Melbourne.

Tonia Todman

I was never brought up to have a career, although I did have ambitions. When I was in my final year at school, doing my leaving certificate, NBN opened in Newcastle, and I thought I was destined for a career in news and current affairs, so I auditioned. My mother made me a wonderful dress, in which I thought I was a million dollars, and they were impressed.

A few days later they rang me and said what a wonderful audition and, by the way, can you sing and dance?

And I said, 'Definitely not. If I am going to read the news, why do I need to sing and dance?'

'We don't want you to read the news,' they said, 'we want you to compere *Young Talent Time*.'

And with that I collapsed on the floor. *Young Talent Time* (or *Swallow's Juniors* as it was called then) was not really what I had in mind, but I did one series, much against my better judgement, and everybody else's, needless to say, but the die was cast. I never ever forgot that experience. I had such fun. I really enjoyed it, and I should have followed my heart, but my parents and boyfriend all thought if I pursued that career I would be led astray.

I married at twenty, after declining the offer of a scholarship to go to university, and worked until I had my first child at twenty-five.

I tended to think of myself as the last of the good wife and mother brigade – the very idea sends shivers down my spine now, of course – and I really only started to work at home to supplement the family income. My husband was still studying, and I wanted to pull my weight. We had similar ideals about the way we wanted to live, and to achieve our aims we needed more money, so I turned to what I could do, and that was sewing.

I started by working for *Vogue* patterns. For ten years I was able to work at home while my children were young. I just went step by step towards where I am now.

When television reared its head again in my forties, I was creative editor of *Mode Made*, a lifestyle magazine. Channel Ten was starting a morning program and rang me to see if I thought it would be possible to transfer my magazine ideas to television. It took me about a nanosecond to say, 'Of course.' They didn't know that I had had any television experience, and I didn't know what they wanted, but I knew I could do something.

Once again I was given a screen test, and a new career was formed. But I also maintained my journalism. I never really had just one job. It may be my innermost insecurities coming out, but I never put all my eggs in one basket, as far as work is concerned. I taught textiles to secondary students, I manufactured and exported, I worked on radio, I wrote twenty or so books on craft and decorating, you name it, and I have always had magazine articles on the go.

I have to say that I did notice some changes as I went through my menopause, but it is hard to be specific. I am no less ambitious now than I was as a younger woman. In fact, I am probably more ambitious now than I was ten or even five years ago. But I guess what is working against me now, which is peculiar to the industry I am in, are social forces, because in the public eye a woman gets too old to be of any value.

Interestingly, I was an expert in my area before I got into television and was valued for what is up here in my head, but my public persona became a face on television. I think I am the oldest woman appearing on television regularly and that's alarming – not only for me, but for women in general. If I were a man I would be called wise, but for a woman it is a bit of a problem. There is no language for it.

But I am not going to let it get the better of me. It is something that I am fighting. It is not so much the lack of opportunity but a kind of negativity, and I have had to work around it. I have decided to achieve what I want by trying another route. My website – toniatodman.com – may just do everything that television did for me, or it might help me to do more in that medium. Happily, I still have television work, but I'd like to do more in the form that I want, that I design.

My mother was a very reserved woman, and it was all I could do to find out about my menstrual cycle at the time let alone reproduction or menopause. I am not even aware of my mother going through menopause. It was not something we ever discussed. I was probably oblivious to it. So I had no role model there.

I breezed through life thinking, Well, I guess it has to happen to me at some stage, but I am not anticipating it, I am not sitting back waiting. It is interesting that the symptoms – I haven't really had symptoms, but let's call them that – have been annoying rather than anything else. They have been an irritation, and I wish they would hurry up and go away.

I approached the menopause with a practical outlook, as I approach most things in life. It was inevitable that it would happen to me, but it was never going to be any source of regret for me. I was past having children. There was no need to mourn, no grief. If I had been a single woman who had never had children, I might have looked at it differently, but I had joyously fulfilled my role as a mother. Sure, I wish I had had more children, but I calmly decided that when menopause happens it happens. If it is a nuisance, then I will do something about it, but I tended to ignore it. And I have sailed through it.

Certainly, things happened to me and I thought, Oh, this must be menopause, but it was not enough to interfere in any way. I guess I noticed mood swings more than anything – I would notice that I was feeling fragile, or unusually feisty, or a little depressed. But there were no prolonged periods of any of these moods.

Mood swings certainly affected me. I am not naïve enough to say that they didn't, but in my case, and it is a pretty old-fashioned story, if I was feeling out of sorts, or that the world was against me, or that nothing I was doing was right, or whatever, then I just got on and got busy with something. It was the best cure I knew. Or I'd go to a funny movie. Laughter, in any form, cured it.

It is one of the tricks that nature plays on us: when we hit menopause we are at a time when there are huge changes in our lives. We have the empty nest syndrome, ageing parents, husbands who are restless, the male menopause, children who are making career choices and probably getting married themselves. This hits you all at once, when you are least equipped to deal with it, when you are less competent or decisive than you'd like to be. I think nature is pretty unfair; she got that wrong. You would be much more able to cope when you are thirty-five or forty than when you're fifty or fifty-five. I sometimes wonder if I could have done it better. The impulses are still there, the energy is still there, but sometimes I reflect on the choices I made, or the things I did.

But going through menopause has not really affected my daily activities to any great extent. I dealt with things as best I could, knowing that whatever is happening is happening for a number of reasons but not necessarily because it is menopause.

I must say I feel rather smug these days, feeling that I am one up on younger people in my field because I have the knowledge that comes with age, and the life skills that young people are not taught today, such as cooking and furnishing a house, that in my time were a normal part of education, or your mother or grandmother taught you. Now there are three generations who have been highly educated but who have possibly never learnt to sew or cook. Grandma, or Auntie, is probably sailing the world with her boyfriend, and the last thing she wants to do is teach the grandchildren to sew or cook.

As far as my credibility is concerned, I am old enough for young people to think that I must know what I am talking about and the older people know I am old enough to have been taught the right way. My audience is across the board: young, old, in-between and, delightfully, the gays like me! A dear gay friend once told me that I was the woman he'd like to be – I don't know what you want to make of that one, but it's a huge compliment. I guess the moral here is that if you are going to be in the public eye, at least impart some knowledge that is valuable.

I am conscious of growing older but in the case of my career, potential problems may not materialise if television networks start to be more amenable to older people (read 'women') appearing on television. There is a glimmer of hope because the networks appear to be recognising that the baby boomers are their biggest and wealthiest audience. So they surely can't fight us for much longer. If I was in America it wouldn't be a problem; it seems to be a particular Australian difficulty.

I have never been seriously overweight. I am tall and large-framed, but I am carrying more weight that I want to, probably because I have been neglecting my regular walking exercise. About three or four years ago I lost of lot of weight just by being diligent about taking daily walks. I am now back at the weight I was when I was in my late twenties, and I am a size fourteen, but I have this size twelve wardrobe there smiling at me, and I would like to get back to being a size twelve. I know how to lose the weight. It is simply a matter of being disciplined enough to get back into that routine.

Somehow I am too busy and too tired by the end of the day to set off on a walk. I am a night walker, and I usually do a lot of work at night. I find I do my most productive work at night, when the phone stops ringing and I can think without interruption. I do know how to fix my weight – and will do just that!

I have always enjoyed cooking and cooking in a healthy way. My biggest problem, if there is one, about my diet is that I eat too much. I have a very healthy appetite. I wish I didn't, but there you go. I am very much aware of nutrition, what's needed to keep people going properly. I am probably eating less red meat and more vegetables than I ever did, and I'm probably drinking less alcohol – and I can go two weeks without a red wine, though I do like a good red.

When I can relax and enjoy myself, I can drink half a bottle of red wine with a meal and be quite happy about it. But that is very rare. I don't mix alcohol with work. If I am working, I never drink. I have to say that when you stop drinking alcohol you do feel better. But that doesn't mark me as a wowser. My husband has a wonderful cellar, and I enjoy helping him enjoy it.

I am finding that I am rather forgetful these days, but again it is my own fault, and the result of being so busy. I run a diary, but my schedule changes sometimes hour by hour, so diaries are impossible, and I keep everything in my head, and that's a problem. I can tell you what I am doing next week, but I have forgotten what I have done this week. Once it is done it is finished.

Nature seems to be saying, 'Slow down, you are getting a bit silly,' but I don't see why I should. I don't want to. I would like to sleep for eight hours a night, but that is a luxury for me. I am beginning to sleep less and less, but that's because my head is full of ideas and plans. I don't have an assistant or a secretary, and there is only so much a human brain can take in each day. I think I am at that point where I am dealing with too much information.

I looked forward to the menopause being over and done with, finished, done. I used to say, 'Why can't it happen earlier? Why can't you push a button and that's it?' I was terribly disappointed when my doctor told me only a couple of years ago that he thought I was still extremely fertile and I thought, Oh, surely you are wrong. Can't you make some sort of changes there? Don't be quite so happy telling me this because it's not a good thing to hear. I don't mourn the passing of my fertility or my periods at all.

I think I've become rather reflective during my menopause because I have reached that point in my life where there are changes, not only physical ones. All the things that life has fastened us to start to move around – as I said, parents, children, work. And having suffered the loss of my mother, I must now contemplate my own life span. That bothers me most because I start to see that I have a certain number of years left and I still haven't done half of what I want to do.

In some ways reflection is a source of frustration for me, and when I re-evaluate what I am doing, I find it is hard to make decisions that I am sure I will be comfortable with in the next ten years. I don't know where I will be in ten years or so.

I hope to live well and laugh a lot. I sometimes think, and this is a bit of a sad way of seeing it, that as I lie there dying what will I regret not doing. So I make lists. What are the books I want to read, what do I want to write, where do I want to travel, what do I want to achieve? Okay you might live in the house you think you want to live in, you might have the way of life that you have planned, but there is always more you want to do. The world is always out there. I think it is very unfair that you only get one go at life.

I think it is another sneaky trick of nature that it is not until you get to fifty or so that you can afford to think, Well, I spent all those years doing things for other people, what am I going to do for me? There are some awful imbalances in the way life is dealt out to you.

One of the other things that happens when you get to fifty is that you become more philosophical and certainly more forgiving of children. I see the restraints that were put on me as a child and as a young woman – the compulsion to be married, to have a family, to gain respectability, to make a mark as a member of the community – and I think there is nothing wrong with any of that. But there is a lot more to life than that.

I look on the exploits of my children, who are in their mid-twenties – my father, bless him, thinks they are wasting their time and should be married with children by now, with a mortgage and whatever – and I envy them. I look back now on the narrow life that I lived at their age and think they would be mad to be tied down. I want them to live as much of life as happily as they can until they really want to settle down. They should decide. It should not be me or society that makes the choice for them.

Patience has set in – maybe that's nature helping you to be patient with grandchildren, or maybe I'm starting that process towards being the most tolerant granny in the world.

I have regular medical checkups – pap smears and mammograms – and think you are mad if you don't have them. There is no excuse. I had a curette a few years ago because, for the first time in my life, I had an abnormal pap smear. There was no serious concern, but it was enough to frighten the daylights out of me. Mammograms, I think, are the most hideous examinations. It really hurts when you get squashed between those two plates. But they are good for your peace of mind.

When I last visited my doctor, he suggested I go on to hormone replacement. But he didn't really say why he thought it would be good for me. He just asked me a few questions, and I think it was probably easier for him to prescribe it and see what the results were.

I have been to a gynaecologist, who gave me a stack of literature about the menopause, which was frankly repetitive and didn't really tell me anything I didn't know.

If I have to have anything, it will be natural before I consider hormones. I have several friends who are on hormone replacement and think it is the best thing they have ever done. They say, 'Oh, sanity has come. I feel terrific, I'm this, that, and the other.' I don't want to muck around with nature unless I have to. I am aware that I have symptoms, I don't call them problems, but they are not unbearable. I believe I can control my mood swings by being aware and treating this naturally. I just don't see any point at this stage in taking the risk of mucking around with my system. Whatever problems nature dishes out, whatever she wants, I will deal with it, as and when.

Chapter Eight
Osteoporosis

What is osteoporosis? How decreasing oestrogen increases bone loss. Why osteoporosis affects people as they age. Oestrogen and vitamin D. Helping the body to absorb calcium. The importance of protein in the diet and exercise. How is bone mass measured? Treatments for low bone mass: exercise, calcium supplements, hormone replacement therapy, bisphosphonates, and their side effects, other treaments including Raloxifone.

Osteoporosis is a bone disorder characterised by a reduction in the density of the bone and a reduction in its strength. A significant proportion of calcified bone is lost, and there is a breakdown in its supporting 'struts'. As a result, there is an increase in the risk of a fracture occurring with minimal trauma.

In the last twenty to thirty years, as a result of the ageing of the population, osteoporosis has become an important public health issue. Osteoporosis is one of the most common musculoskeletal (muscle and bone) disorders in the elderly. Although it affects elderly women more often than others, it is also a relatively common disorder in men.

When they reach menopause, many women are worried about the risk of developing osteoporosis either because their elderly relatives have suffered from the deformities associated with vertebral or spinal fractures, or because they have had hip fractures. The rounding of the spine is called 'Dowager's hump', despite men with several vertebral fractures displaying a similar rounded profile.

Osteoporosis is defined as 'a systemic disease characterised by low bone mass and microarchitectural deterioration (breakdown in the structure) of bone tissue, with a consequent increase in bone fragility and a susceptibility to fracture risk'.

Many people with osteoporosis are unaware that they have it. There may be no symptoms until a fracture occurs after a minor fall. It is often detected by chance when an X-ray is taken for some other reason. Probably the most common reason will be if a patient complains of back pain. The cause of the back pain could be a fracture of one or more spinal vertebrae, but often the cause is either muscular pain or osteoarthritis around the bones of the spine.

A great deal of bone mass needs to be lost before an ordinary X-ray of the spine or other bones detects it. Possibly about 30 per cent of bone will have been lost. A bone density scan will show a person's risk of developing osteoporosis.

The World Health Organization has defined osteoporosis in relationship to bone mineral density measurements. There is an increasing risk of fracture with decreasing bone density. Thus osteoporosis is defined as a bone density of more than 2.5 standard deviations below the young adult value. This is equivalent, in lay terms, to about 30 to 35 per cent below a young adult bone density value. Bone density measurement predicts future fracture risk in the same way that blood pressure is a predictor for future stroke risk, or serum cholesterol level predicts heart disease risk.

The greatest problem caused by osteoporosis is that of fractures, with the most common fracture sites being the spine, hip and wrist. Fracture risk is related to low bone density and bone strength, and to the risk of falls, particularly in the elderly.

It has been predicted that over the next twenty-five years there will be an increase of about 83 per cent in the number of people in hospital as a result of hip fractures. This will incur high medical costs to our community. The mortality rate associated with hip fractures is about 20 per cent in elderly men and women. Vertebral spine fractures can cause severe and incapacitating deformity, and wrist fractures can cause some morbidity, with, usually, a temporary decrease in the quality of life.

Osteoporosis is one of the most common causes of serious illness in Australia and other countries where the population is ageing.

Osteoporosis is either a primary or a secondary condition. Primary osteoporosis includes postmenopausal osteoporosis associated with oestrogen deficiency. It also includes the bone loss associated with ageing. Secondary osteoporosis is loss of bone due to the effects of an underlying cause on the absorption of calcium into the body or the laying down of calcium in the bone. Secondary osteoporosis may be associated with cancer, such as multiple myeloma, drug use, including cortisone, hyperparathyroidism (an overactive parathyroid gland) and hyperthyroidism (an overactive thyroid gland). Secondary osteoporosis can also be caused by the excessive breakdown of bone.

> 'It is one of the tricks that nature plays on us: when we hit menopause we are at a time when there are huge changes in our lives . . . This hits you all at once, when you are least equipped to deal with it, when you are less competent or decisive than you'd like to be. '
>
> TONIA TODMAN

Once menopause is reached, the production of oestrogen from the ovaries falls to very low levels. In women, oestrogen is one of the most important hormones that builds up and maintains healthy, well-calcified bones. Primary osteoporosis starts in the perimenopausal period. There can be a rapid loss of bone mass for the first five to ten years after menopause. Rates of loss vary from 3 to 6 per cent each year during this time.

The trabecular, or more porous bone of the vertebral spine, is the principal area of bone loss during this time. This is related to the greater rate of bone turnover in this area. Bone turnover is the process of bone building up and bone breaking down.

Bone is very active throughout life. It is in a constant state of remodelling. With loss of the strong hormonal effect of oestrogen at menopause, there is a greater rate of breaking down than building up, which results in an overall loss of calcified bone. Connections between calcified areas of bone are lost, so that the bone becomes thinner and weaker. Vertebral or spinal fractures are relatively common in women in their sixties.

In elderly men, both oestrogen and testosterone levels are lower. Oestrogen is as important as testosterone in maintaining bone mass in ageing men, and oestrogen deficiency may also contribute to continuous bone loss in ageing men.

Bone loss related to ageing is slower and more gradual than the bone loss related to oestrogen deficiency.

Part of the reason for bone loss occurring with age is the decrease in the activity of the bone substances that promote the building up of bone. The other cause of osteoporosis developing with ageing is the decline in the production of vitamin D in the body and a decrease in the absorption of calcium from the bowel.

The parathyroid glands are four little glands that are located behind the thyroid gland in the front of the neck. Parathyroid hormone is an important hormone that helps to maintain the level of calcium in the blood stream. As well as its importance in bone, calcium has other important functions in the body. It must be maintained at a fairly stable level in the blood. If calcium is not being absorbed into the body, the parathyroid hormone starts breaking down bone to help build up the level in the blood. This results in bone loss.

Where there is calcium wasting, dietary calcium intake needs to be increased to maintain calcium balance within bone. Fractures tend to occur in the hip, spine and ribs in elderly people.

About 50 per cent of women over the age of fifty, will sustain an osteoporotic fracture. The most frequent early fractures are wrist and vertebral fractures, followed by hip fractures in elderly women. About a third of women will experience a hip fracture by the time they are eighty-five. A significant factor for hip fractures in the elderly, other than low bone mass, is falls. Poor muscle strength, postural instability, decreased visual acuity, and side effects of drugs such as those that lower blood pressure or drugs that are used as sedatives may contribute to falls.

Reduction in bone mass, or osteoporosis, is the major risk factor for fracture. Measuring bone mass is therefore the most useful guide to assessing future risk of fracture. But bone mass measurement only determines the *quantity* of bone not the *quality* of bone.

Peak bone mass, or the maximum level that bone builds up to, occurs around the late teens to early twenties. Genetic or inherited factors account for about 75 per cent of the population variance in peak bone mass. Twin and family studies have been important in identifying the role of genetic factors. There have been several genes identified that play a role in building up bone. These include the vitamin D gene receptor and the oestrogen receptor gene.

In adolescence, factors that influence the attainment of peak bone mass include dietary calcium, vitamin D, hormonal factors such as delayed puberty, and hypogonadism. Hypogonadism is underactive sex hormone glands – the ovary in women and the testes in men. Physical activity and concurrent medical illnesses such as coeliac disease also affect peak bone mass.

Some adolescents may suffer from conditions such as asthma requiring high, prolonged oral doses of cortisone. They may suffer from anorexia nervosa, which is often associated with significant weight loss. This can affect menstruation. Prolonged low oestrogen levels associated with amenorrhoea (absence of menstruation) or oligomenorrhoea (infrequent periods) can contribute to bone loss in young women. Some adolescent girls are involved in the intensive exercise programs of elite athletes or ballet dancers. Exercise by itself can cause a usually temporary loss of periods and therefore low oestrogen levels. Strenuous physical exercise can delay puberty because of the effects of the exercise on hormones that are produced within the brain. These hormones are needed, in turn, to stimulate the ovary to produce oestrogen. Lack of sufficient production of these hormones means that the bone is not stimulated to thicken and grow.

In both men and women, there is a gradual decline in bone mass from around thirty-five years of age. The rate of loss with ageing is about 1 per cent a year. Risk of fracture is therefore dependent on both the maximum level of the peak bone mass and the rate of subsequent bone loss. From menopause onwards, there is an accelerated loss of bone for about five to ten years.

Epidemiological studies show that an increase of peak bone mass by 10 per cent would potentially decrease fracture rates by half. Adolescent males have an increase in bone size and cortical thickness as a result of a more prolonged maturation phase compared to adolescent females.

After menopause 20 to 25 per cent of bone mass can be lost in the first five to ten years. An increase in bone resorption (breaking down of bone) is the primary mechanism resulting in bone loss. Even in elderly men and women there can be a substantial degree of bone loss. It is therefore still important to treat older men and women with appropriate therapies to prevent further bone loss and fractures.

Some of the risk factors for osteoporosis are family history, malabsorptive syndromes, premature menopause, hyperpara-thyroidism, low calcium intake, and hyperthyroidism, immobilisation or excessive exercise, a small build, low body weight, smoking, excessive alcohol intake, prolonged amenorrhoea (absence of periods), prolonged treatment with cortisone, such as those used in the treatment of asthma, chronic liver disease, and chronic renal disease.

About 75 per cent of osteoporosis may be due to a genetic predisposition. Risk factors only identify about 65 per cent of those who have osteoporosis. Bone density measurement is the only definitive tool to specifically diagnose osteoporosis.

It is important for women at menopause to address poor diet, low levels of calcium intake, smoking and any unnecessary drug use that may contribute to the loss related to oestrogen deficiency. Physical activity is also important in preventing excessive bone loss.

Smoking is one of the most potent factors affecting risk of osteoporosis. Smokers tend to be thinner than non-smokers, and smoking also appears to lower oestrogen levels by increasing the metabolism of oestrogen. Smokers may also exercise less and have a higher intake of alcohol. A high intake of protein and sodium in the diet, high caffeine intake and alcohol in excessive amounts may adversely affect bone density.

A lifelong low intake of calcium may reduce bone density. The recommended minimal daily intake of calcium is 500 mg. Dietary levels of calcium in premenopausal women should be 800 to 1,000 mg daily, and postmenopausal women should maintain a daily intake of 1,000 to 1,500 mg.

Elderly men and women are often deficient in calcium as a result of eating small amounts of food, the decreased intestinal absorption of calcium, lack of exposure to sunlight, and the reduced capacity of the body to produce vitamin D. These people should be encouraged to eat more dairy foods and to take some calcium supplements. The reduction in appetite and the overall calorie intake in elderly people often makes it difficult for them to achieve optimum nutrition.

A person's vitamin D intake can also affect their osteoporosis risk levels.

The recommended daily intake of vitamin D is 400 international units. This dose will also prevent osteomalacia, another bone condition that can lead to fractures. It occurs when the levels of vitamin D in the body are very low. The bone is weak in this condition because the normal structure of bone is distorted from the lack of vitamin D. Vitamin D3 (cholecalciferol) is derived from the diet and from the skin by the ultraviolet irradiation of 7-dehydrocholesterol, the form of vitamin D that is found in the skin. Vitamin D is then converted to the more active form in the liver. The resulting product, 25-hydroxylated vitamin D, is the main form of vitamin D that is routinely measured in laboratory testing. It provides an index of the nutritional value of vitamin D.

Plasma levels of vitamin D decrease by 50 per cent with age in men and women. Vitamin D2 (ergocalciferol) is used to supplement the diet. It is commercially available as Ostelin 1,000 international units. In women who do not have very low levels of vitamin D, a supplement containing lower levels of vitamin D combined with calcium is sufficient.

The second step in the metabolism of vitamin D is its further conversion in the kidney, mainly to 1, 25-dihydroxyvitamin D3, or calcitriol. Production of calcitriol is enhanced by the action of hormones such as oestradiol, prolactin and growth hormone. Vitamin D2 and D3 are similar in their actions and metabolism.

The main action of vitamin D is to increase the intestinal or gut absorption of calcium and phosphate. It increases the availability of calcium and phosphate for mineralisation, or laying down of bone. With ageing, there is a decline in kidney function and therefore a decline in the production of calcitriol or vitamin D.

Osteomalacia is common in people in institutions and probably results from the combination of a lack of exposure to sunlight with decreased production of vitamin D within the body and poor nutrition.

Another nutritional deficiency that may affect bone health is a poor dietary intake of protein, particularly in the elderly. Poor nutrition is common in elderly people who have a hip fracture. Lean-muscle wasting is associated with an increase in the propensity to fall. Reduction in food intake, and in particular protein intake, can be the result of physical and mental illnesses.

Physical activity is important in developing peak bone mass. Regular exercise helps maintain bone mass and muscle strength. An increase in lean-muscle mass should be taken into account when measuring bone mass changes as a result of exercise.

The risk factors for fracture include a bone mineral density measurement of about 35 per cent below the young adult value. One vertebral fracture increases the risk of further fracture by five times, but two or more vertebral fractures leads to twelve times the risk of further fracture.

The most common diagnostic techniques used for osteoporosis are radiology, DEXA scans, QCT scans and ultrasound. Plain X-ray is useful for defining or diagnosing fractures, but it is not a very sensitive measure of bone loss.

Osteoporosis will only become apparent on a plain X-ray if the bone mass is decreased by about 30 to 50 per cent. A decrease of 20 per cent in any of the heights of one or more vertebrae compared to other vertebrae is regarded as an osteoporotic fracture. The vertebrae of the spine are squashed or compressed (called a crush fracture). Plain X-rays are also used to diagnose malignancy, osteoarthritis or other bone pathologies. Calcification of the aorta can also be detected. A DEXA scan is the gold-standard diagnostic technique for determining if osteoporosis is present. Two areas are commonly assessed: the femoral neck (hip) and the lumbar spine (lower). Usually the average bone density of the values between lumbar vertebrae 2 and lumber vertebrae 4 are measured – that is, the lower part of the spine.

Measurement at the lumbar spine can be less accurate in the elderly than in younger patients because the scan detects other areas of calcification, such as a calcified aorta (the large blood vessel that supplies blood to the lower body), osteoarthritic bone on the vertebrae or facet joints (these are the bony joints that protrude from the vertebrae and help support the spine).

Osteoarthritis is quite different from osteoporosis, and is discussed in the chapter on arthritis. Osteoarthritis is characterised by extra bone growth around joint surfaces, whereas osteoporosis is a thinning within the structure of the bone. Osteoarthritis is very common in the spine of many people from age fifty onwards. Extra bone can give a falsely higher bone-density reading. If there is a significant difference between the spine bone density and the hip bone density, the hip result is considered the most reliable indicator of degree of bone loss. Measurement at the hip is a good indication of whether osteoporosis is present in the hip as well as the rest of the body. This technique is associated with low radiation and is precise and reproducible.

A QCT scan measures bone density at the spine only and is associated with much higher levels of radiation.

Quantitative ultrasound of the heel has been introduced in the last few years. It measures the fragility of bone rather than the bone density. Quantitative ultrasound does not involve ionising radiation and may provide information about the structure of bone other than bone mass. This technique is still undergoing assessment and may be more useful in determining risk of fracture in the future.

These techniques confirm the diagnosis, review the efficacy of treatment (whether the treatment is working in building up bone and preventing fractures) and the efficacy in high-risk patients (those with pre-existing fractures), in patients with co-existing medical problems such as those suffering from malabsorption, chronic liver or renal disease, rheumatoid arthritis, patients on steroids and people who have thyrotoxicosis, and to monitor the treatment – a follow-up scan is usually ordered after two years, but if there is a significant change in therapy, then the patient will be assessed again after one year.

In someone who has a bone density a great deal below others of the same age, we might do other investigations.

The by-products of bone formation and resorption can be useful additional measures of the rate of bone turnover before and after initiating treatment. These are special tests often used in research, but they may also be used in clinical practice occasionally.

Bone markers could potentially be used to monitor bone mass response to therapy. This technique will give earlier information than bone density measurements.

Treatment aims to reduce further bone loss, increase bone mineral density and prevent further fractures. Management includes preventing falls, encouraging regular weight-bearing and muscle-strengthening exercises, avoiding drugs that aggravate bone loss or increase the potential for the risk of falls, and improving overall nutrition and adequate calcium and vitamin D levels. Drug therapy may be necessary to prevent further bone loss and fractures.

Elderly people who fall are at great risk of breaking their bones. Drugs, diseases and the environment all contribute. Drugs include hypnotics, tranquillisers, alcohol, antihypertensives, hypoglycemics and diuretics. Impaired vision, neurological conditions such as Parkinson's disease, and slippery surfaces, loose rugs, wires and stairs are all potential causes of increased risk of falls.

Older people should be encouraged to participate in regular exercise, including exercises to enhance muscle coordination and strength.

Extra calcium is the most common non-hormone replacement therapy for treating osteoporosis. Many studies show that calcium supplements (more than 1 gram per day) will slow bone loss to a small degree in women, with or without fractures, after menopause. Calcium appears to reduce bone turnover. It seems likely that there is a small increase in blood calcium levels, resulting in a decrease in parathyroid hormone. High levels of parathyroid hormone tend to break down bone – therefore it is important to keep its level low.

A study by Chapuy in 1992 in France, supplementing the diet with calcium and vitamin D in elderly patients in nursing homes, showed that they suffered a significant decrease in the number of hip fractures. This may have been because nursing home patients are not exposed to sunlight and also being elderly they don't tend to form as much of the active type of vitamin D in their bodies. In other words they may have had vitamin D deficiency.

There are small differences in the absorption of over-the-counter calcium in the different proprietary preparations, but this is unlikely to be significant in treatment. The elemental content (that is, the amount that is actually available to be absorbed in the bowel) of calcium varies with each calcium product. It is important to divide the daily dose as the maximum absorption at any one time is from the equivalent of a 600 milligram tablet, and the calcium supplement can be taken with meals.

Calcium carbonate contains 40 per cent of elemental calcium, whereas calcium phosphate contains 31 per cent, calcium lactate has 13 per cent and calcium gluconate contains just 9 per cent. The differences in the amount available, however, are probably not significant – as long as the dose from any calcium source is in the range 1,200 to 1,500 mg per day. This of course will ideally include food sources of calcium – particularly dairy foods or calcium-fortified soya products. The risks of using recommended doses of calcium supplements with or without vitamin D are negligible in otherwise healthy people. Common side effects include bloating, flatulence and constipation.

Calcium supplements should not be given to patients with excessively high levels of calcium in the urine. This is because calcium stones can form in the kidney. They should also be avoided in patients taking normal drug doses of drugs such as Calcitriol or Rocaltrol.

Postmenopausal women have a relative deficiency of oestrogen. This leads to a loss of bone mass in the postmenopausal years. Bone loss is relatively rapid in the first five to ten years after menopause. Some women will reach menopause with a bone mass that is already reduced. This reduced bone mass may be caused by genetic factors, lack of periods (especially for more than six months), or drugs such as cortisone. Hormone replacement therapy prevents the bone loss in the early postmenopausal years and treatment with it greatly reduces the extent of the loss.

Studies that have looked at women who have used hormone replacement in the past have shown that there is a reduction by 60 per cent in the risk of fractures in the wrist and vertebrae and a reduction by 40 per cent in the risk of fractures of the hip.

Several randomised controlled trials show that there is an increase in bone density if hormone replacement therapy is taken, but there are only a few short-term studies showing a reduction in the rates of vertebral fractures. There are no randomised, controlled trials showing a reduction in the rate of hip fractures. Some women will be concerned about the long-term use of oestrogen and the possibility of a small increase in the risk of breast cancer that this brings.

Observational studies have provided the most information on the overall risks and benefits of hormone replacement therapy. The problem with these studies is that women who elect to take hormone replacement therapy are known to differ in many ways from women who do not. Women who take it are generally better educated, exercise more frequently and have lower morbidity and mortality rates.

There are a number of long-term studies of the use of hormone replacement therapy taking place, including the Women's Health Initiative in the US and the WISDOM study in Europe, and it is hoped that these studies will clarify some of the concerns about hormone replacement therapy use and the benefits of its long-term use.

The five most commonly used bisphosphonates are etidronate, alendronate, clodronate, pamidronate and risedronate. Bisphosphonates have an action specifically on bone, they are not hormones. Over the next few years, however, many new bisphosphonates will become available. The bisphosphonates work to prevent the breakdown of bone that occurs after menopause.

The effects of different bisphosphonates on bone resorption or breakdown varies. Bisphosphonates are generally poorly absorbed from the gastrointestinal tract, particularly when taken with foods containing calcium. They should be taken after an overnight fast and 30 to 60 minutes before food. The bisphosphonates, whether taken orally or injected, are quickly taken up by bone. Bisphosphonates have a very long half-life, probably even several years, and for this reason may have a long duration of effect.

The bisphosphonates that have been used in Australia to prevent osteoporosis include alendronate (Fosamax), pamidronate (Aredia), etidronate (Didrocal) and risedronate (Actonel). They have been used in postmenopausal women and patients on cortisone. All bisphosphonates prevent bone loss over one to two years, or longer.

Increases of 2 to 10 per cent in bone mineral density have been noted in the first year of treatment, depending on the site – that is, hip or spine – measured.

Alendronate has been used in randomised, controlled trials. The Fracture Intervention trial (FIT 2) studied 4,432 women who had osteoporosis but no fractures at the beginning of the study over four years. There was a decrease in vertebral fractures in those women who were in the active treatment group compared with women who were in the inactive or placebo group by 50 per cent.

In the FIT 1 trial over three years, alendronate reduced the rate of vertebral fractures in 2,027 women with osteoporosis and baseline fractures by 40 to 50 per cent. In the FIT 1 study, 50 per cent fewer hip fractures occurred in the treatment group compared with placebo. The dose of alendronate that is most appropriate for osteoporosis is 10 mg a day.

Etidronate, a bisphosphonate, is used as a cyclical regime as continuous treatment results in adverse mineralisation of bone. Its intermittent use is more effective in preventing breakdown of bone. For fourteen days every three months, 400 mg is given daily. During the interval, 1,250 mg of calcium is given daily. Etidronate has been shown in small trials to reduce the rate of fractures of the vertebrae.

Risedronate is a new bisphosphonate that has been shown to be effective in reducing vertebral fractures and hip fractures in postmenopausal women. At a dose of 5 mg a day it reduced the rate of fractures in the spine by 41 per cent over three years. In the first year, the reduction in the number of fractures was 65 per cent.

The most common side effects of the bisphosphonates are gastrointestinal. Alendronate has been associated with ulceration of the oesophagus if the medication is not taken as directed with a full glass of water on an empty stomach and with patients remaining upright for half an hour. If gastrointestinal symptoms do occur early in treatment, they may settle if the medication is stopped for one to two days and then reintroduced.

Intranasal salmon calcitonin (Calcitonin) has been studied in a two-year trial. Bone mass density increased by 3 per cent with a small decrease in the number of fractures of the vertebrae. It is not widely used in practice in Australia.

Fluoride was shown to increase bone mass density by 10 per cent in the first year of use. This increase, however, was not reflected in an increase in bone strength. Fracture rates did not differ between treatment and control groups.

Calcitriol, or 1, 25 dihydroxyvitamin D, both increases the absorption of calcium from the intestine and raises the serum calcium level. As a result, it reduces parathyroid hormone, which then reduces bone formation and breakdown. The response to treatment has been mixed. Some studies have shown large increases in bone density, but this may be due to the healing of co-existing osteomalacia in patients deficient in vitamin D. Osteomalacia is an abnormality of bone caused by vitamin D deficiency. It causes weak bones in a similar way to osteoporosis.

A New Zealand study (Tilyard, 1992) showed a difference in the number of new vertebral fractures. This randomised, but open, study of over 600 postmenopausal women showed a difference in the rate of new vertebral fractures in the second year of treatment. The difference in the rate of fractures, however, was due to an increase in the rate of fractures in the control group taking calcium alone.

Raloxifene is the first of a group of selective oestrogen receptor modulators (SERMS) to be released on the market for treatment of osteoporosis. It has been approved for use in postmenopausal women who have established osteoporosis with fractures arising from minor falls or lifting heavy objects. Raloxifene is related to Tamoxifen, a drug used in the treatment of breast cancer, which has been shown to have oestrogen-like effects on the skeleton and lipoproteins (blood cholesterol and triglycerides).

Raloxifene has no effect on the breast or uterus. It has been shown at a dose of 60 mg to increase bone mass density by 2.4 per cent in the lumbar spine and total hip at two years. In a large placebo-controlled trial (the MORE study) of 7,700 postmenopausal women with osteoporosis with or without vertebral fractures at the beginning of the study, the number of new vertebral fractures at two years was reduced by 50 per cent. All patients were given 500 mg of calcium and vitamin D 400 international units daily. Raloxifene reduces total and low-density lipoprotein (LDL) cholesterol levels, but has no effect on high-density lipoprotein (HDL) cholesterol levels and triglyceride levels. Tryglyceride is another fat that can be abnormal in the blood.

Analyses of several studies of 10 000 women followed over three and a half years with yearly mammograms showed a reduction in the relative risk of breast cancer of 0.42, a 56 per cent reduction with Raloxifene use. Raloxifene use has an increased risk of venous thrombosis and pulmonary embolism that is similar to hormone replacement therapy and Tamoxifen. The risk is greatest in the first six months of therapy. The risk is twenty-eight in 100 000 patients a year. Other side effects include hot flushes and leg cramps.

Raloxifene should only be given to postmenopausal women, not premenopausal women. Two other SERMS – idoxifene and levormeloxifene – are being trialled.

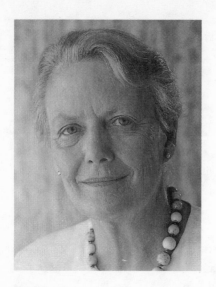

Jan Wade studied Law at Melbourne University as well as taking out the degree of Bachelor of Arts. After graduating she travelled overseas where she worked in England for two years as a school teacher. She then became a tutor at Melbourne University. She continued her career as a solicitor until 1967, when she began work in the Parliamentary Counsel's office, becoming an Assistant Chief Parliamentary Counsel in 1978. Between 1979 and 1985 she was Commissioner for Corporate Affairs. In 1985 she was appointed President of the Equal Opportunity Board, and remained in this position until 1988 when she was elected Member for Kew in a by-election for the Victorian government. She was re-elected in 1988, 1992 and 1996 and retired from Parliament in 1999. During her period as Member for Kew, she held many distinguished parliamentary positions culminating in the position of Attorney General, Minister for Women's Affairs and Minister for Fair Trading from 1992 to 1999. She is currently Distinguished Visiting Professor, Victoria University, and writes a monthly column for the *Australian Financial Review*.

Jan Wade

I can't really remember what age I was at menopause. I've been wracking my brains. I'm sixty-three now, and I went into Parliament in 1988 – twelve years ago, so I would have been fifty-one. I think it was around about that time.

When I was at university I saw myself getting married and having children and not working, but for various reasons I stayed in the workforce after I had children, mostly because I needed the money.

After I left school I did law at Melbourne University. When I finished my course, I went overseas to England for two years as people did then. It was the thing to do. I was married over there. I came back, tried to get a job as a solicitor and couldn't because I was married and all the firms said, 'You'll be having children, and we want someone permanent.'

My husband, on the other hand, had no trouble getting a job as a solicitor. He went through with me and in fact his results weren't as good as mine. So I thought, If I can't get a job, I might as well have a baby. I was thinking along those lines when I was offered a job as a tutor by Sir Zelman Cowen at Melbourne University, which I took. About a month after that I realised I was pregnant. Zelman was very good about it, and I stayed on and kept working for another couple of years and had a couple more children.

By that stage, I think I had become a workaholic. Despite having the children, I felt it was my responsibility to earn a reasonable percentage of the family income, and I just kept working. I think I'm even having difficulty with that as a retired person. When people ask me to do things, I find it difficult to refuse. I think that has come about from juggling five children – four children of my own and a step-daughter – and a job. I just kept powering along regardless.

I wouldn't really change anything. But it has been quite hard work. A lot of young women who have worked for me over recent years who are thinking about having children have asked me how I have managed work and children. It was difficult. I'm very pleased to see that law firms now are not only employing married women but being much more flexible about it – letting them work part-time, or from home, and so on.

I think in a way I've sacrificed my social life, but I'm catching up with it a bit now. It was either work or the children when I was younger, and there wasn't much social life other than work-associated social life.

From 1983 to 1987, when I was about fifty, and before my menopause, I had what I consider now, in retrospect, to be something like yuppie flu or chronic fatigue syndrome. It went on for about four years. I got terribly tired, I'd ache all over, and I felt frightened to drive the car. My response at the time was to keep working. I just about went out of my mind with it. I went to several doctors and eventually to a specialist who was a general physician.

I would suddenly feel overwhelmingly tired and have aches across my lower rib cage and in my wrists and at the back of my neck, and I felt generally stiff. It would last for several days and then pass off. It felt like glandular fever, which I did have when I was twenty-two, the year I did my articles.

The physician did all these tests and nothing showed up and he decided I was suffering from depression. He said I should come back and see him in six months, but I gave it away then. I'd seen so many doctors with no result and I thought I really would be depressed if I continued. Interestingly, each of the doctors I went to said, 'Well, what are you working for? You don't need to work. Why don't you give it away?' At that stage I was Commissioner for Corporate Affairs, and then I was President of the Equal Opportunity Board. I'm sure they would never say that to a man.

One of the reasons I continued working when I married Peter Wade in 1978 was that I had four children and he had one daughter, and I felt it was not appropriate for him to support all of my children. I felt that I should continue working, and I was enjoying my career.

I'm not sure when I look back whether I was suffering from some kind of viral infection or whether I was having menopausal symptoms or hormonal changes. Whatever it was, it wore off around about 1988. The only thing I did have around that time was migraines. I had those when I first went into Parliament. I can remember that. I think they started in 1985 when I was on an overseas trip and they stopped some time after I went into Parliament. I also remember having hot flushes and sweats around the same time. But they were not particularly worrying.

I tried hormone therapy twice, and both times I gave it away. I was so pleased not to have periods anymore. I quite welcomed that aspect of it. I thought it was fantastic. And also the hormone replacement used to make me come out in pimples, so I gave it away for that reason as well. Some people see hormone replacement as the key to eternal youth, but I can do without pimples.

I don't much like the thought of getting older, but I like being alive. Getting older hasn't really affected me very much in terms of the way I feel.

At the moment, I feel extremely fit, even though I have just had breast cancer. I was looking at my armpit one day, and I just saw two tiny little lumps, one about the size of a pea. You could actually see them. It was breast cancer, but it wasn't in the breast.

I went along to see the doctor, and everyone said, 'No, it's perfectly all right, it won't be anything.'

But when they took one of the little lumps out to have a look it turned out to be cancer.

I had a mammogram the year before, and of course it didn't show up in the mammogram because it was not in my breast but in the axillary tissue. So, I've had chemotherapy and radiotherapy.

Apart from that I've felt the fittest I've ever felt, probably because I'm not working, and working always made me feel a bit tired. Now I've got a brand new head of hair, the best hair I've had in my whole life.

I went through divorce, in the 1970s, and I found then that I had to re-evaluate my entire life. I had the major responsibility for four children so I thought very carefully before I remarried.

The next time I re-evaluated my life was when I went into Parliament because that was a big change too. At that stage we had two children still at school.

If anyone is going into Parliament they really need to think carefully about it. Particularly Federal Parliament, which I think is very hard on any life. In making a decision to retire I thought that the Kennett government was going to continue. I didn't think we'd be in opposition. I thought I'd have another four years of trying to do things that I thought were important.

On the other hand, I really felt that I had worked so hard for forty years without much play that I wanted to have some time for myself. My father died when he was thinking about retiring at fifty-nine, and I think that has really had an effect on me. There is a history of heart disease on both sides of the family. My little brother had a quadruple by-pass in 1999, and I thought I'd get out while the going was good. Cancer was not on the agenda at all.

My husband was semi-retired. He'd made a decision about a year before that he was going to semi-retire. I thought that if he's going to be able to holiday a bit more, I don't want to be sitting here in the Victorian Parliament. With our five children we've both had to work quite hard to do what we've wanted to do. For the first time, we're free in financial terms. We've now been married for about twenty-three years. Most of it, however, has been pretty full of people and work.

In the next twenty to thirty years I'm hoping to become proficient in golf. I want to continue to work, but not too much. I'm trying to improve my language skills. I'm trying to become proficient in French at the moment. Like so many other people, I've always wanted to draw and paint. I haven't managed to do that yet, because I feel that I have to be in a more relaxed mode than I am in now. It's funny, all my life I've been doing things that I think I'm quite good at. Now I'm trying to tackle sport and painting, activities that are more challenging, because I feel I do not have a lot of talent. I'd really like to travel, however not in the way I have travelled in recent years. This was usually two days here and two days there. I'd like to travel somewhere and spend a couple of months there.

I'm trying to slow my life down. One of the things I feel is that my life has gone past too quickly. I thought that retiring might have slowed it down, but it hasn't.

I try to walk a reasonable distance every day. I don't actually achieve that. I don't follow any special diet. I've always eaten very sensibly, I think. Although, now, I am trying to eat more fruit and vegetables. I'm still having at least one glass of wine with dinner, and I like red wine. I've never been a heavy drinker. Since I've been concerned about my heart in the last year or so, I've cut down on cheese. I used to eat a lot of cheese, and chocolate.

I think moderation is a good thing. I don't go overboard either way. I don't try to be too hard or too soft on myself. I've probably been hard on myself when I was working – perhaps conscientious is a better word. I've tried to do everything. I've tried to eat properly. I've tried to bring up the children properly. I've tried to carry out my work as well as I could.

Ultimately, I do believe you can have it all. You can have an interesting and challenging career, a good marriage, and you can have children. I had my first child in my early twenties and the last one when I was thirty-three. They have been a very important part of my life which would have been poorer without any one of them. My husband, Peter, has been my greatest supporter at home and during the more challenging parts of my career. Our family is expanding with daughters-in-law and sons-in-law and five grandchildren with a sixth about to come. There's nothing I regret about any of it. I've had a fabulous life, absolutely fabulous.

Chapter Nine
Cardiovascular disease in postmenopausal women

Why women are not safe from heart disease. How oestrogen might prevent the onset of heart disease. Cholesterol levels. Weight gain. Diabetes. The studies into oestrogen and progesterone treatment to prevent heart disease. Other drugs for lowering lipid levels. The results of three studies into the effects of hormone replacement therapy in preventing heart disease. Things you can do to reduce your risk of heart disease. More on diabetes in relation to heart disease.

Before menopause, heart attacks and strokes are uncommon in women. Those at most risk of heart disease in their thirties and forties are women who have a strong family history of high blood fats, who smoke, have very high, uncontrolled blood pressure, or suffer from diabetes.

The protective effects of oestrogen in the premenopausal years have long been considered to be the reason why women don't have a high incidence of heart disease at the same ages as men.

However, heart disease is just as common in women as it is in men. Death rates from heart disease in women are very high. Heart disease is about ten times more common as a cause of death than breast cancer. But a large proportion of women believe that they are more likely to die of cancer than heart disease or stroke, and breast cancer seems to be the cancer that they most fear. Deaths from heart attacks and strokes tend to occur in women who are over the age of seventy. About 50 per cent of women will die of cardiovascular disease (heart attacks and strokes).

Around the age of fifty, however, the death rates from heart disease and breast cancer are about equal. But death rates from any cause in women in their fifties are low. Most women die when they are elderly. The average life expectancy for women is around eighty years.

Compared to men, women tend to visit their doctor more often and are likely to use more medications, which may suggest that they pay more attention to preventive health than do men. We are all aware how difficult it is to get the men in our lives to visit the doctor for a check-up.

It is not entirely clear if oestrogen is the main factor in preventing heart disease in women in the premenopausal years. There is a steady rise in the incidence of heart attacks as women age after menopause. Oestrogen may play a role in maintaining a more favourable balance in the levels of the blood fats, in the distribution of body fat, and in the metabolism of blood sugars and insulin levels.

Looking at statistics on body mass index, obesity and general increasing weight in women from their forties onwards, there is a definite increase in the slope of the curve. Women, overall, are not as overweight as men when they are in their thirties and forties. But they start to catch up to men in their forties and fifties in both body weight and heart disease rates.

We do know that, after menopause, when there are lower levels of oestrogen, there is a rise in total blood cholesterol levels, and that the balance of the different types of cholesterol becomes less favourable. The levels of the 'good' or more protective type of cholesterol, high-density lipoprotein (HDLc), and the 'bad' cholesterol, low-density lipoprotein (LDLc), change after menopause.

There is a tendency for HDLc to decrease and for LDLc to increase. Ideally, total cholesterol levels should be less than 5.5. HDLc should be more than 1.2 and LDLc should be less than 3.5. (These figures are measured in pmol per litre and may vary a little from one laboratory to another.)

If you are having your cholesterol measured, always ask for the HDLc and LDLc to be measured. Some women have a cholesterol level greater than 5.5, but if this is due to a level of LDLc less than 3.5 and a HDLc greater than 2.0, then the balance is favourable and they should not be concerned about their total cholesterol level.

Another blood fat that is important to measure, particularly in women with a strong family history of heart disease at an early age, or who are diabetic, is the triglyceride level. Women with diabetes often have an increase in this blood fat as well as high levels of total cholesterol and LDLc and lower levels of HDLc. These abnormal levels of blood fats explain part of the increase in risk of heart disease for women with diabetes at any age.

'I view myself as a well-informed person, but I found I was surprisingly ignorant of a number of health-related issues. I had never spent any time thinking about menopause, I suppose because there seemed to be more interesting things to think about.'

BARBARA CHAMPION

After menopause, the distribution of body fat changes. There is a tendency to put on weight around the abdomen or midriff. There is about a 10 per cent shift in body weight to this area, a cause of great concern in many women who become frustrated when their clothes no longer fit them. This change in body fat may be related to the hormonal changes and also to the general tendency to gain weight.

Abdominal weight is not as healthy as weight on the hips, although it is often hard to convince most women of this, particularly young women who would like to have no hips. A 'pear-shaped' figure is associated with a lower risk of diabetes and heart disease than an 'apple-shaped' figure. If you observe overweight men, you will notice that they tend to gain weight in the abdomen – the so-called beer-pot. These men often have a less favourable distribution of body fat, which may explain their higher risk of heart disease at a younger age. As previously mentioned, men seem to gain weight at an earlier age than women.

After menopause, diabetes is much more common in women than in men of the same age. Oestrogen plays a role in the use of blood sugars in muscular tissues. Muscles do not use sugars as efficiently in postmenopausal women. The pancreas is the organ in the body that produces insulin. If blood sugar levels are high, or there is an insensitivity or resistance to normal levels of insulin in the tissues such as muscles, then the pancreas produces more and more insulin if it can.

The pancreas produces more insulin to encourage the muscles to take up sugars from the blood stream. High levels of insulin are not healthy. Although it is important for body function to improve the use of sugars by muscles, high levels of insulin also cause an increase in the amount of body fat being deposited, particularly around the abdomen.

There are two types of diabetes.

In one form of diabetes (type 1), there is a deficiency of insulin production from the pancreas. This type tends to occur in young people. There appears to be a genetic susceptibility in this group, and other events, such as a viral infection that results in destruction of the special B-cells in the pancreas, may lead to a deficiency in insulin.

In the second type of diabetes (type 2), which is much more common, the body can produce adequate levels of insulin if body weight is normal. This form of diabetes tends to occur in overweight or obese people who are putting their pancreas under excessive strain. The pancreas produces higher and higher levels of insulin.

The role that oestrogen replacement therapy plays in the prevention of heart disease and diabetes is still being evaluated. Many research studies have compared women who have used oestrogen replacement therapy with women who have not. These studies – called observational studies – have compared the rates of heart disease and strokes in each group. Researchers tend to look at what women have done in the past. These studies, however, have some limitations. Some characteristics in the group of women who take hormone replacement therapy may be different from the group that does not take it. This could lead to a biased result.

One explanation of why these studies may be biased is that healthier women (that is, those women who are keen to reduce their risk of heart disease) may be more inclined to take oestrogen replacement therapy. These women may actually have a low risk of heart disease already, or are adopting a way of living that reduces their risk as well as taking oestrogen replacement therapy.

These studies do not always take into account other factors that may be associated with heart disease, including obesity, diabetes, hypertension, smoking, high cholesterol levels and a family history of heart disease at an early age.

Overall, the observational studies have shown a 50 per cent reduction in mortality in women who take oestrogen replacement therapy compared with women who do not take it. Some of the studies have also suggested that oestrogen replacement therapy is particularly beneficial for women who have had heart disease.

Ideally, we would like to confirm what has been 'observed' with more reliable evidence. The most reliable evidence is from studies known as randomised, placebo-controlled, double-blind trials. These studies compare two groups of women over a period of time. Each woman in the research study is allocated either to a group that contains a drug or other therapy or to a group that has an inactive or placebo treatment. Neither the subject nor the doctor knows whether the placebo or the active treatment is being taken.

In assessing whether a treatment works or not, it is important to account for the 'placebo effect'. This is the belief that there will be an effect simply from taking the medication or undergoing treatment. The placebo response may be significant, particularly if there is a belief that treatment or medication will be beneficial. The placebo response can be as high as 40 per cent, meaning that 40 per cent of people taking an inactive treatment receive some benefit from it. Any improvement as a result of the active treatment must be over and above the placebo effect to show that the treatment works.

There are some long-term research studies being conducted to assess the benefits of oestrogen therapy, and oestrogen plus progesterone therapy, in the prevention of heart disease.

Most of our information on heart-disease risk and hormone replacement therapy use is based on studies in the US, where oestrogen was used for many years in postmenopausal women without the addition of progestins. (Women who have had a hysterectomy do not need to use progestins.) In these early studies, oestrogen was used alone, even in women who had not had a hysterectomy.

After several years of oestrogen-only use in women who had not had a hysterectomy, there was an increase in the incidence of cancer of the uterus. The lining of the uterus, called the endometrium, becomes excessively thickened and is more prone to cancerous cells developing without the protective balance of progestins.

'I have a tremendous group of girlfriends and we talk about these things together very easily – we laugh about them. When people close to you are going through the same experiences, you don't feel so different, alienated or depressed.'

ELAINE CANTY

Oestrogen-alone use may have a more protective effect against heart disease than when it is combined with progestins. Some progestins, however, appear to have more helpful effects than others when used with oestrogens. Norethisterone acetate, for example, found in some combination preparations of hormone replacement therapy, may prevent the increase in triglyceride levels that occurs with oral oestrogens. This may be of benefit in women with diabetes, although more research needs to be done in this area.

Progestins that are more like the progesterone that the ovary produces before menopause, for example, micronised progesterone (not yet available in Australia), may be more beneficial than the other progestins. Some progestins appear to counter the benefits that oestrogen provides in lowering cholesterol levels in postmenopausal women. The effects, however, are small and whether these effects are significant in long-term use will only be determined by properly controlled studies over an extended period.

Oral oestrogens tend to lower cholesterol levels (in the range of 10 to 15 per cent), increase HDLc levels to a similar degree and lower LDLc levels. Oral oestrogens, however, tend to increase triglyceride levels. This may be important in diabetic or other women who already have high triglyceride levels.

Transdermal oestrogens, patches and gels tend to have the same effects as oral oestrogens on total cholesterol, HDLc and LDLc, but not to quite the same extent. Transdermal oestrogens do not, however, increase triglyceride levels and may be of benefit to women who have high triglyceride levels.

Much research is underway in the laboratory on the effects that oestrogens may have in reducing the fatty build-up in blood vessels (called atherosclerosis) and in the ways that oestrogen opens up (or dilates) narrow, constricted blood vessels.

Some research has shown that oestrogen may work in the same way, or as effectively, as nitroglycerine tablets, which have been used for many years to treat angina. The long-term benefits these have on the risk of heart disease in postmenopausal women is still to be determined.

Other research is analysing whether oestrogen is as effective as other drugs that lower cholesterol. Blood fat or 'lipid-lowering' medications are effective in their ability to reduce death from heart attack in men, but it can only be surmised that they are as effective in women, because women were not recruited for study when these research studies were undertaken. The researchers only evaluated the effects in men.

Heart disease in women has been somewhat neglected in many areas, including work on the prevention of further heart disease in the treatment of women who have had heart attacks. Presumably, this is because men appeared to have a higher rate of death from heart disease than women. It appeared that relatively young men died of heart disease whereas women died when they were much older. With the increasing rate of diabetes in postmenopausal women and the general tendency for increasing obesity in western societies, heart disease in relatively young postmenopausal women may become more of a problem.

Short-term studies show that the lipid-lowering drugs (affecting both cholesterol and triglyceride) have similar effects in lowering cholesterol and triglyceride levels in women as in men. Women, therefore, should also be treated with lipid-lowering drugs if they have high blood fat levels.

The Nurses Health Study is a longitudinal study of hormone therapy use and heart disease that involves a large group of women (59 337) who have participated since 1976. Some women have taken hormone replacement therapy and others have not. It has investigated hormone therapy use and the risk of cardiovascular disease, including the risk of pulmonary embolism (clots to the lung).

In this study, various issues about hormone replacement use and cardiovascular disease have been evaluated. The results suggest that women who have few or none of the risk factors for heart disease do not gain any benefit from using hormone replacement in reducing their risk of heart disease.

The researchers also found that the survival benefit diminishes with longer duration of the use of hormone replacement therapy. This may be because its longer use (more than ten years) is associated with a possible, but small, increased risk of breast cancer.

The study also found that the relative risk of pulmonary embolism in users of hormone replacement therapy is twice that of non-users. In general, the occurrence of pulmonary embolism is very small, occurring at a rate of one in five thousand women.

There have been more recent randomised, double-blind, placebo-controlled trials using hormone replacement therapy such as the PEPI trial (the Postmenopausal Estrogen/Progestin Interventions trial), which used unopposed oestrogen – the use of oestrogen without progestin – in women with a uterus – and three oestrogen/progestin regimes. The investigators compared the effects of hormone replacement therapy on cholesterol levels in the hormone replacement therapy group and the placebo group.

Healthy postmenopausal women aged forty-five to sixty-four years participated in this study. The trial was conducted over three years and evaluated four endpoints or outcomes: high-density lipoprotein cholesterol (HDLc), systolic blood pressure, blood insulin and fibrinogen, a blood-clotting factor.

The study concluded that oestrogen alone, or in combination with a progestin, improves blood fats and lowers fibrinogen levels without detectable long-term effects on insulin levels or blood pressure. This study did show a benefit of oestrogen and oestrogen combined with progestins on cholesterol levels. The study, however, was only over three years and focused on healthy women. The findings of the study do not tell us whether this reduction in cholesterol level will lead to a reduction in heart disease in the long term or whether it is applicable to women who already have heart disease.

'Every year in your life is a bonus; it doesn't matter whether you are old or young. You get up in the morning and you are lucky to be alive, lucky to be doing the things you like doing. You take the bat and ball and keep playing. That's what life is all about.'

LILLIAN FRANK

In 1998, a randomised, blinded, placebo-controlled trial called the HERS (the Heart and Estrogen/Progestin Replacement) study was published. It was a secondary prevention trial that evaluated the use of hormone replacement therapy in women with pre-existing heart disease. It was looking to see whether hormone replacement therapy used in women who had experienced a heart attack would reduce their risk of having another episode. As mentioned earlier, observational studies had already indicated a reduction in mortality in women with pre-existing heart disease and hormone replacement therapy use.

The problem with observational studies, particularly case-controlled studies, is that there are biases and confounding factors that may not be accounted for in the design of the study, or in the analysis of the results. These factors may strongly influence the outcome of the study either favourably or in a negative way.

This research trial included 2,763 women with coronary artery disease who were younger than eighty years, postmenopausal and still had their uterus. The average age of the women was 66.7 years. The length of the study was averaged at 4.1 years. The regimes used were 0.625 mg of conjugated equine oestrogens plus 2.5 mg of medoxy-progesterone acetate, or placebo.

The researchers were mainly trying to see whether there was an increase in the occurrence of non-fatal heart attacks, or death from a heart attack when women were on hormone replacement therapy. More minor issues were other cardiovascular outcomes. The researchers wanted to see whether more operations were needed to clear blocked heart blood vessels (called angioplasty), whether there were continuing episodes of chest pain (angina), heart failure, strokes or transient ischaemic attacks (small strokes) and blockage of the blood vessels in the legs. All deaths from any cause were also considered in the study.

The results showed that, overall, there were no significant differences at the end of four years in death rates and the rate of heart attacks between the women who took hormone replacement therapy and the women who did not.

In the hormone group, 172 women had a heart attack or died from a heart attack, as did 176 women in the placebo group.

The lack of an overall effect came about despite a net 11 per cent decrease in LDLc and 10 per cent higher HDLc, two favourable changes in blood fats. There was a trend for more cardiovascular events, such as thrombosis (blood clots) or heart attacks in the first year, and fewer in years four and five.

More women in the hormone treatment group experienced an increased rate of venous thromboembolic events (blood clots) and gallbladder disease.

The investigators concluded, or advised, that, based on the results, they did not recommend starting hormone replacement therapy for secondary prevention of cardiovascular disease. Women who are not on hormone replacement therapy and who have heart disease already should not start it.

If women are already receiving treatment with hormone replacement therapy, however, it would be appropriate to continue treatment, given the favourable patterns after several years of therapy.

As the results of the study were contrary to what had been expected, based on the observational studies, various opinions and explanations have been put forward. These criticised the type of hormone replacement therapy used in the study, although it is the most common regime or combination of oestrogen and progestin used by postmenopausal women in the US, and questioned whether the study should have been conducted over a longer period since longer use of hormone replacement therapy had begun to show a benefit in reducing the death from heart attacks.

'I approached the menopause with a practical outlook, as I approach most things in life. It was inevitable that it would happen to me, but it was never going to be any source of regret for me.'

TONIA TODMAN

At this stage, the study is still the best evidence that we have on giving women who already have heart disease hormone replacement therapy.

Whether it may be of benefit in the prevention of heart disease is being tested in two very big, randomised, controlled studies, one called the Women's Health Initiative being conducted in the US, and the WISDOM study, being conducted in Europe. The results of the WHI will be available in 2007.

It is very important for postmenopausal women to reduce their risk factors for heart disease. Unfortunately, little can be done about your family history, but if members of your family have suffered early death from heart disease, this may increase your desire to reduce all other risk factors.

Not smoking is definitely beneficial in reducing your risk of suffering from heart disease. Smoking is also a strong risk factor for osteoporosis and lung cancer, which is increasing as a cause of death in women.

Reducing cholesterol and triglyceride levels has also been shown to reduce heart disease death rates, but it is important to reduce LDLc as well as the total cholesterol level. This can be done initially by reducing the amount of saturated fats in your diet and by combining this with thirty to forty minutes of daily exercise, such as brisk walking.

If this initial strategy is not effective – it may be difficult for women who have an inherited cholesterol problem – then consider taking one of the lipid-lowering medications. The aim is to achieve a LDLc of around 2.5, a HDLc of greater than 1.2 and a triglyceride level less than 2.0. The triglyceride level should be measured after an overnight fast because a recent meal or alcohol can suggest an increase when there is not a true problem.

Reducing fats in the diet, and reducing daily alcohol and calorie intake can decrease triglycerides.

Maintaining weight in the healthy weight range is also important. These days we evaluate body fat distribution (the waist–hip ratio), which should be less than 0.9, and the body mass index.

You can measure your waist–hip ratio by dividing your waist measurement by your hip measurement. You can measure your body mass index by dividing your weight in kilograms by the square of your height in metres. There are many charts available that will indicate your body mass index at a glance. The healthy range for body mass index is twenty to twenty-five. Over twenty-five and up to thirty is in the overweight range and over thirty is in the obese range.

Another important risk factor is high blood pressure, or hypertension. Untreated hypertension is a strong risk factor for strokes and heart attacks. If improving factors such as diet and lack of physical activity is not effective in reducing blood pressure to the normal range, then drug treatment may be needed. There is very good evidence from randomised, controlled studies that reducing blood pressure to the normal range reduces the death rate from heart attacks and strokes. Even given the side effects of some medications, reducing blood pressure to the normal range improves overall quality of life and well-being.

Postmenopausal women with diabetes have an increased risk of premature death from heart disease. They need to be very conscious of maintaining strict control of their diabetes as well as the other risk factors for heart disease. As yet, there is insufficient evidence regarding the use of hormone replacement therapy in diabetic women. There is some evidence that low doses of oestrogen may improve the metabolism and use of blood sugars in diabetic women, thus helping to lower high insulin levels.

Whether hormone replacement provides an additional benefit to all these strategies for reducing cardiovascular disease in postmenopausal women is still to be determined from further research.

Diabetes is more common in postmenopausal women than it is in men of the same age. Women aged between fifty-five and sixty-four have 64 per cent greater prevalence of diabetes than men. Non-insulin dependent diabetes (type 2) is the most common form of diabetes in this age group. Risk factors for diabetes include a history of gestational diabetes, a family history of diabetes, age and obesity. Women who have features of polycystic ovary syndrome are also at risk.

The hormonal changes associated with menopause, particularly the changes in oestrogen levels, increase the susceptibility to type 2 or non-insulin-dependent diabetes (NIDD).

There is an increase in insulin resistance and reduced insulin sensitivity predominantly in muscles. This results in hyper-insulinaemia, or an increase in blood insulin levels. Insulin resistance is aggravated by physical inactivity, upper abdominal obesity, hyperandrogenism, ageing, thiazide diuretics and cortisone. High insulin levels stimulate lipid or fat storage, alter lipoproteins (decrease HDL and increase LDL) and increase ovarian androgen or testosterone production.

Compared with men who have diabetes, women with diabetes have higher triglyceride levels and lower HDL levels. Both disturbances are strong risk factors for cardiovascular disease.

Oestrogen deficiency, associated with menopause, results in an increase in total cholesterol, a decrease in HDLc and an increase in triglyceride levels. Menopause contributes to the adverse lipoprotein profile already present in diabetic women and increases the high risk of cardiovascular disease. Diabetes increases the risk of cardiovascular disease by five to six times.

In premenopausal women, the oral contraceptive pill with high doses of oestrogen results in impaired glucose tolerance, that is, blood sugars are increased. However, the low physiological doses of oestrogen in hormone replacement therapy (usually equivalent to the low levels of oestrogen in the early phase of the menstrual cycle) appear to improve carbohydrate metabolism.

There are few recent studies that have evaluated the effects of oestrogen alone, or oestrogen with progestins, in diabetic women. There are some studies that have investigated glucose and insulin metabolism in non-diabetic postmenopausal women, for example, the PEPI trial. Oestrogen in low doses has a favourable effect on glucose and insulin metabolism. In oestrogen/progestin regimes, some progestins may be more favourable than others, for example, norethisterone acetate and dyhydrogesterone.

While we await the outcome of further studies on hormone replacement use in diabetic women, it is important for postmenopausal diabetic patients to address the various strategies for controlling their diabetes and reducing their risk of cardiovascular disease. This should include controlling weight and reducing obesity through a structured diet and exercise program. Exercise should be at the level of at least thirty to forty minutes each day, six days a week. Diabetic patients are strongly advised to stop smoking, reduce hyperlipidaemia, that is, high cholesterol and triglyceride levels (drug therapy may be needed for this) and control hypertension. Recent trials in diabetic patients with hypertension indicate that strict blood pressure control is very important in reducing the death rate from cardiovascular disease.

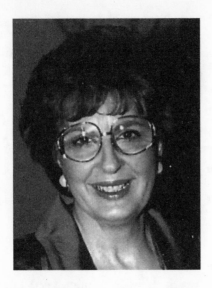

Diana Abruzzi is the founder and a director of the International Women's Federation of Commerce and Industry and is currently its first Executive Chair. Diana is well known for advancing new ideas and strategies, and for her contribution both nationally and internationally as a public speaker on issues important to women. In this capacity she has greatly helped the development of small business, international trade and the general economic advancement of women in business. Diana is also involved in directorships of Fusco Investments Pty Ltd and Fusco Plant Food Company, and is a founder/director/publisher of the *Business Women's Review* magazine. Currently Diana is the Vice-President and founding member of the Confederation Women's Business Council-APEC Economies where she has been given the task of forming an Australian Women's Bank.

Diana Abruzzi

During the years leading up to menopause I was very confident, entrepreneurial, with incredible energy. Nothing daunted me, I loved challenges that stretched my abilities. I had a real zest for living. I travelled around the world, for business and pleasure. I met a number of amazing people while travelling, some of whom have remained personal friends over the years.

The first indication I had that things were not as they should be was when I started to feel very disoriented. There was a distinct sense of feeling not all together. I was very tired and found it hard to concentrate.

To make matters worse, menopause was never discussed or talked about in my era. Women just soldiered on, suffering in silence with no real support or understanding from husbands or doctors – who in many ways were even more ignorant on these matters, with no idea in how to handle these changes affecting women. In fact women took a lot of criticism, and up until recently male doctors on the whole treated them with very little sympathy.

A very dear friend of mine went through a terrible time. She felt she was dying, and the doctors kept telling her to go away, it was all in her head. I asked her what the sensation was like. She said she couldn't explain it, only that there was this overpowering sensation of herself dying and the hardest part was fighting these sensations.

It was this same dear friend who introduced me to the hormone replacement patch. I often think, If men had gone through menopause a cure would have been found a long time ago.

So here I was feeling all these strange effects going on in my body, not knowing a thing about it. One day I happened to be speaking with my mother, and I shared with her the strangeness I was feeling and how I was not having my periods as frequently.

I might add, that was the best thing to come out of menopause. That and not having to worry about fertility. I had three boys in three years, of whom I am very proud, and I think after that I felt I had done my bit. Although I do regret not having a daughter. I know there are women in Europe who are having babies in their sixties – but who wants to start having children at sixty? And I think it's not fair on the children because not only is there a huge generation gap they can also lose their parents at the very age they need them most. Having said that, I have just taken on a fifteen-year-old stepson, which has brought a whole lot of new challenges into my life. But since I have always had quite a heart for the young it doesn't daunt me.

Anyway, back to that conversation with my mother. I can still remember her response today. She said, 'Don't worry. You have started your change of life. I sailed through it, there is nothing to worry about.'

Menopause, I found, affects different women differently. Women like my mother never noticed any changes; other women experience extreme changes as I did. I have also heard women who have their tubes tied can experience even greater effects through menopause, how true this is I am not sure.

Women who have spent most of their lives looking after husbands and children also seem to experience extreme effects while going through menopause. Perhaps this is brought on by the emotional downturn in their lives, as children become more independent and with husbands still very involved in their work. It's what they call the empty nest syndrome.

Women today are so lucky, they have literature available to them, clinics to assist them and medical breakthroughs, such as hormone replacement. At first I was a bit sceptical about hormone replacement in the pill form, as I had heard it could have extreme side effects. When they brought out the patch I went straight on to it and have been using it now for over nine years. The stabilising effect was wonderful and I have never looked back.

In regard to my business life, before I went on the patch, everything seemed to go on as normal. Only now looking back I realise I must have been really pushing myself throughout that period, because I remember an extreme lack of energy and concentration. I just wouldn't accept what was happening and wouldn't give in to it. Something that did come out of that period was the necessity for taking notes on everything. This has stood me in good stead over the subsequent years, especially when you are trying to run several things at the same time.

One of the effects of menopause which really put my health at risk was my massive weight gain. Even though my diet had not changed, I was really packing on the weight and I felt physically uncomfortable with it. It wasn't until I was introduced to Jennie Craig that I really began to tackle the problem, and in under a year, I had lost over four stone, making me feel younger and more alive. I was not only on the diet but also exercising and drinking heaps of water and that I believe is so vital as you get older.

This period was also a time to re-evaluate my life, where was I going, and what I wanted to achieve with the later part of my life. It wasn't menopause that caused this need to re-evaluate. Five months earlier I had gone for a yearly pap smear test only to find that I had pre-cancer and would need to have major surgery. Without this I don't think I would have considered re-evaluating my life, I was too busy getting on with things.

I would really like to emphasise at this point the need for all women not to neglect these tests. Without my test, and immediate action taken by the doctors, I would have been dead within six months. Today I am fine, with a clear bill of health, but this is what really pulled me up to start thinking about my life.

When I was in my twenties, I thought by the time I was fifty I would probably be retired. I am now sixty-one and far from being retired. I had no idea that at this age I would be undertaking far more than I had in all my years leading up to this time. I was in fact increasing my workload, not decreasing it. With my health intact, I believe I will still be going strong at eighty.

I remarried at fifty, after twelve years on my own. This was a major change to my life right in the middle of going through menopause, but I never really gave it much thought, I think because I was so happy.

The changes I made are really basic, once I realised they had to be made. The first thing was to keep myself from getting too overloaded with commitments as I have always done in the past. I never make appointments now before 10 o'clock if I can help it. I also now have a fully equipped office at home and only go into my office when I have to. I have found this to be very convenient, as I deal with a lot of international business which is usually done late at night.

I would like to spend more time with my husband and family. With both our hectic schedules this is sometimes impossible, but we are making the effort now. My youngest son and I often catch up for meetings over breakfast, as we are working on a couple of projects together. At least it takes us out of the office environment. The rest of the family I usually catch up with on Sunday at church where we have four generations of our family attending.

I have always been self motivated and have always been my own boss. I have always had a keen interest in the economic development of women. Being on my own for twelve years and responsible for my three boys gave me a great insight into the needs of women and the obstacles they face in business. This led me to start up the International Women's Federation of Commerce and Industry which I have remained committed to. I would like to play an even greater role in bringing about changes for women in business within developed and undeveloped countries. I would like to see more action and less talk.

Chapter Ten
Arthritis

What is osteoarthritis? What parts of the body it is likely to affect. Treatments: pain relief, exercise, anti-inflammatory drugs and creams, 'Synvisc', joint replacement, alternative therapies. The importance of weight control in the prevention of arthritis. Other forms of arthritis: lupus, rheumatoid arthritis, fibromyalgia. The role of hormone replacement therapy in the prevention of arthritis.

Arthritis is a common disease in women, particularly in the peri-menopausal and postmenopausal age group. Osteoarthritis is the most frequently occurring arthritis in women. Hormonal, genetic and environmental forces seem to play roles in its development.

Osteoarthritis often starts in the perimenopausal years. It is at least three times more common in women than in men. In the past it was called 'menopausal arthritis'.

Osteoarthritis affects the joints, specifically, the hyaline articular cartilage, which covers the joint surfaces. Cartilage coats the bony surfaces of the joints, providing a soft cushioning to the bone surfaces. This cartilage allows the bony ends to move smoothly against each other. Wearing down of the protective cartilage results in narrowing and often distortion of the joints. The destruction of the cartilage surface is also associated with extra abnormal bony growths around the joints. Many women notice that they start to develop small lumps over the joints of their fingers, particularly the joints nearest the nails. These little nodules are called Heberden's nodes.

The terms 'osteoarthritis' and 'osteoporosis' are often confused. They are quite different conditions linked by the common term 'osteo', which refers to bone. Osteoarthritis affects the joints. Osteoporosisis is a thinning of the bones from loss of the calcified area of bone.

With osteoporosis, the long bones of the arms and legs are particularly affected, as are the bones in the spine. There is a general loss of calcium in the body, but some bones are more prone to fracture than others. Thinning of the bones results in an increased risk of fracture.

Women who are prone to osteoarthritis seem to be less likely to develop osteoporosis, although the two conditions can occur together. Some women may have osteoporosis of the vertebrae and osteoarthritis of the joints, called the 'facet joints', around the spine.

More than 45 per cent of women over the age of sixty-five have symptoms related to arthritis. Osteoarthritis causes pain and varying degrees of disability. If we X-rayed everyone over the age of sixty-five, about 70 per cent would have arthritis.

The most common joints affected by osteoarthritis in women are the hands, hips, knees and spine. 'Primary generalised arthritis' is the term given to the arthritis that occurs predominately in perimenopausal women. It is the 'nodal' form of arthritis that causes the lumpy growths on the fingers.

Women with nodal arthritis often also develop arthritis of the knee, hip and spine. The cause of this type of osteoarthritis has not been defined, that is, we don't know why it begins. Because it tends to occur around menopause, changing hormones have been considered to be one of the causal factors.

As well as developing the extra little bony growths on the joints, women with osteoarthritis complain of pain, stiffness and swelling of the joints. One joint of the hand that is often the first to give symptoms is at the base of the thumb. Although the joints can become painful and swollen for several months, they may settle down and the function or mobility of the joints of the hand may be quite good despite the bony deformities.

Other symptoms include increasing stiffness after inactivity, loss of the full range of movement of the joint, instability and insecurity, or a feeling of the joint 'giving way'. Sometimes there is a grating sound in the joint. Generally, the joints in osteoarthritis are not swollen or red, but occasionally this can occur.

> 'I decided that now my kids have a life of their own,
>
> I'd better have a life of my own too.'
>
> JANNIE TAY

Osteoarthritis of the hips and knees tends to be a slowly progressive condition. Being overweight can aggravate or increase the likelihood of developing osteoarthritis of the knees and hips. Weak thigh muscles, particularly the quadriceps muscle, the main muscle at the front of the thigh, can contribute to an increased severity of osteoarthritis of the knee.

Previous joint injury can predispose women to the development of osteoarthritis. Trauma to the joints or damage to the supporting ligaments, for example, can predispose a person to osteoarthritis in the hands and knees. Women who have had tears in their crutiate ligaments or menisci (cartilage) of the knee may be at risk of arthritis later in life. All these factors and other unknown or poorly defined factors seem to result in the breaking down of the articular cartilage that covers the bony ends. The normal joint structure and function is gradually destroyed.

Generally, normal recreational activity doesn't increase the risk of osteoarthritis, but elite athletes who train frequently, or for long periods of time, may be at risk of developing arthritis in later life. Deformities of the joints or incorrect alignment of the joints may also increase the occurrence of osteoarthritis.

There is a great deal of research being conducted to identify the factors that lead to the breakdown of the articular cartilage and ultimately to the development of osteoarthritis. A group of drugs that decrease the breakdown of the articular joint cartilage called 'metallo-proteinase inhibitors' are being evaluated in clinical trials in Australia and overseas.

It has been postulated that there is a relationship between osteoarthritis and hormones, particularly oestrogen, on the grounds that osteoarthritis often starts to develop in women in the perimenopausal and early postmenopausal years. Some recent studies have shown that hormone replacement therapy may protect against the development of osteoarthritis in the hand, knees and hip. But further research needs to be done in this area.

Osteoarthritis may be associated with deformity of the joints and extra little bony growths around the joints. Although these changes may be cosmetically bothersome they may not cause any adverse symptoms, and therefore no treatment is necessary.

If there are symptoms of pain, but no inflammation or redness of the joints, the best treatment is simple pain relief with paracetamol. It is generally safe to take up to 4 grams (eight tablets) each day. Paracetamol does not predispose a person to stomach irritation or ulceration. If paracetamol is combined with codeine, there may be more pain relief, but an increase in side effects, such as constipation.

Other simple ways of improving osteoarthritis include exercises, particularly those to strengthen the quadriceps muscle, and weight loss. Protection of the joint by using a walking stick can be helpful. It relieves pressure on the joint and improves stability.

One effective exercise for the quadriceps muscle is to lie on your back with one knee bent, and, keeping the other leg straight, slowly raise the bent knee. Lift it up and down slowly, feeling the muscle in the front of your thigh tighten as you lift.

Some women find that massaging with anti-inflammatory creams is helpful if the joint is painful and red. Stretching and generally keeping the joints flexible and mobile is also important. Hydrotherapy (water exercises) can be useful as this allows joints to move freely without bearing weight.

If the joint is inflamed and very painful, anti-inflammatory drugs (NSAIDs) may be used. As these drugs can irritate the stomach lining, four to five days' use may be all that is needed. They are often used in combination with other drugs that protect the stomach. A new range of drugs, similar in action to the NSAIDs, has been developed that are collectively called 'Cox 2 inhibitors' because they block the enzyme in the stomach that leads to ulceration. When released in the US, they became one of the biggest selling prescribed medications.

Sometimes, local cortisone injections can be effective as a treatment for inflamed, osteoarthritic joints when combined with a local anaesthetic.

Another new treatment called 'Synvisc' has become available for severe osteoarthritis of the knee. This is a natural substance called hyaluronic acid, which provides lubrication within the joints. A referral to a rheumatologist (an arthritis specialist) may be needed to advise on this treatment. Three injections, one week apart, are usually given. Its cost may be around $450, but it will usually provide pain relief for six to eight months and is effective in providing pain relief in two out of three people. The appeal of this treatment is that it can delay the need for a joint replacement operation.

Joint replacement can effectively return mobility and relieve pain from osteoarthritis in many women. The joints of the hand, particularly at the base of the thumb, hip and knee can all be replaced, even in elderly women, and these joint replacements can provide good function for ten years or longer.

Population-based surveys in the US show that 85 per cent of patients with arthritis try alternative therapies, at a cost of 21.1 billion dollars. A study in South Australia found that $621 million is spent on alternative therapies in Australia each year.

Alternative therapies for osteoarthritis include eliminating certain foods from the diet. But there is no substantial evidence that this is effective. Some people also wear copper bracelets.

Substances that have been used as alternative therapies include Zinax (ginger extract), green-lipped mussel, the penny-wort plant, fish oils, chontriotin sulphate (Glucosamine), antioxidants such as vitamin E and C, and celery seeds.

Some of these substances have been evaluated in controlled clinical trials. Zinax was shown to be better than placebo, but less effective than the weakest anti-inflammatory drug. The side effects are unknown. Green-lipped mussel has a weak anti-inflammatory effect, but there is a risk of becoming infected with hepatitis C. There have been no trials using penny-wort.

Fish oils, which contain omega 3 fatty acids, have an anti-inflammatory effect, but high doses are needed, and they are expensive. The side effects include a fishy odour on the breath and an increased tendency to bruising. Eating fish three times each week will give an equivalent benefit.

Chrondroitin sulphate, or Glucosamine, has been used for over twenty years to treat osteoarthritis symptoms. It is the biggest selling over-the-counter medication in the US. Whether medically prescribed or self-prescribed, the costs of treating osteoarthritis are huge for the person and the community.

'Nowadays I think people are so driven by what they do, rather than who they are, that they feel inadequate. A hundred years ago people used to ask about your family and no one was interested in what you did or how rich you were.'

JEANNE PRATT

Herbal treatments have been used by some women and are considered to be effective in controlling arthritic symptoms. Care should be taken in using these treatments because some may contain cortisone, which is effective when used carefully but is not a treatment generally used for osteoarthritis. It may be used by arthritis specialists for other arthritic conditions that produce greater inflammation of the joints than osteoarthritis.

One of the most beneficial strategies that should be adopted by all women to prevent and manage osteoarthritis, whatever their age, is to control weight. Maintaining weight in the healthy weight range is important in the prevention of many diseases, but is particularly beneficial in protecting weight-bearing joints from excessive strain and pressure. Repeated minor damage to these joints may be one of the factors that starts off the process of cartilage breakdown, leading to permanent joint damage. Obesity is one of the strongest risk factors for osteoarthritis, particularly knee osteoarthritis.

Other forms of arthritis occur in women and some of these appear to be associated with hormonal changes. Rheumatoid arthritis occurs in 1 per cent of women, osteoarthritis (hands/knees) in 23 per cent, osteoarthritis (knee) in 3.8 per cent, osteoarthritis (hip) in 1.3 per cent, ankylosing spondylitis (a form of arthritis causing a stiffening of the spine) in 0.1 per cent, gout in 1.0 per cent, psoriatic arthritis (an inflammatory arthritis associated with psoriasis which usually causes a skin rash) in 0.1 per cent, scleroderma in 0.006 per cent, systemic lupus erythematosus (a condition that causes inflammation in many tissues of the body including the joints, lungs, kidneys, lungs and brain) in 0.002 per cent.

Rheumatoid arthritis and systemic lupus erythematosus are more common in younger women of child-bearing age. Osteoarthritis and rheumatoid arthritis tend to affect women in midlife. The most common rheumatic diseases in elderly women are osteoarthritis and osteoporosis. Other arthritic conditions that may also occur in older people include crystal arthritis and polymyalgia rheumatica.

Systemic lupus erythematosus (commonly called lupus) is more common in women in the child-bearing years with a peak age of occurrence around fifteen to twenty-five years. It is an autoimmune disease that affects women in the years when oestrogen levels are higher than they are in older women. It is nine times more common in women than in men. There appears to be an association with abnormal metabolism of oestrogen and low levels of androgens, such as testosterone. Another hormone called prolactin is often high in women with lupus. These hormonal changes may interact with the underlying abnormal immune response to cause the symptoms characteristic of lupus.

Women with lupus who become pregnant need to be carefully monitored during their pregnancy. Low-dose oral contraceptive pills can be used in lupus patients as long as there are no other risk factors present, such as smoking or a tendency to thrombosis. The same precautions need to be taken in women who have lupus and are postmenopausal and want to use hormone replacement therapy. Hormone replacement therapy may be beneficial for women with lupus who are on cortisone, as it may prevent bone loss and reduce the risk of osteoporosis.

Rheumatoid arthritis is a chronic inflammatory condition predominately affecting joints. The cause of rheumatoid arthritis is unknown, but it affects twice as many women as men. The peak ages for the onset of rheumatoid arthritis are forty to fifty years, that is, in the perimenopausal and postmenopausal years. There appears to be a genetic predisposition to the development of rheumatoid arthritis. Genetic factors interact with environmental and hormonal factors. Many researchers have postulated that infective agents such as viruses or bacteria may also play a role.

'As my mother puts it – she's semi-disabled and walks with the aid of two sticks – "The chassis is cracking up but the engine is running beautifully."'

ELAINE CANTY

Epidemiological studies suggest that rheumatoid arthritis symptoms often decrease in pregnancy, but recur or 'flare up' again in the postpartum period. The higher oestrogen levels during pregnancy appear to modulate or alter the immune response or inflammation that occurs in rheumatoid arthritis. This is, in a sense, opposite to the hormonal changes that occur with lupus.

Rheumatoid arthritis is also less common in women who take the oral contraceptive pill, where again oestrogen levels are high. Studies that have investigated the role of hormone replacement therapy in rheumatoid arthritis have not shown any significant effect, either positive or negative, on the disease activity or symptoms. As osteoporosis is more common in women who have rheumatoid arthritis, however, hormone replacement therapy may be beneficial in preventing bone loss in postmenopausal women with the disease.

Fibromyalgia syndrome is seven times more common in women than in men. It has a peak incidence in the ages twenty to fifty. Symptoms of fibromyalgia are common in women around menopause.

Fibromyalgia is characterised by musculoskeletal aches and pains and soft tissue tenderness or hypersensitivity. This increased sensitivity to pressure applied to the skin appears to be related to a lowering of the pain threshold, and women with this condition seem to feel pain more readily. Other common symptoms include fatigue, poor sleeping patterns, waking in the morning feeling unrefreshed, headaches, irritable bowel symptoms and stiffness.

A number of population studies have considered the range of symptoms experienced by women at menopause. These studies seem to show that musculoskeletal symptoms are as prevalent as hot flushes in perimenopausal women. This applies to women in western societies and to women in Asian countries such as Japan. Although there are differences in the prevalence of hot flushes in these countries, the rates at which hot flushes and musculoskeletal symptoms occur in each country is very similar.

Hot flushes and night sweats cause sleep disturbance in women at menopause. It has been postulated that the low oestrogen levels at this time may alter biochemical substances such as serotonin in the brain. Serotonin is an important substance in brain function. It is involved in pathways in the brain that modulate or influence pain perception, sleep and mood.

Hormone replacement therapy may be beneficial in relieving the aches and pains that perimenopausal women experience. Increasing oestrogen levels with hormone replacement therapy improves serotonin levels and, therefore, may increase the pain threshold. Oestrogen therapy also alleviates night sweats and hot flushes, so the quality of sleep improves. The mild depressive symptoms that some women experience at this time may also improve with oestrogen therapy.

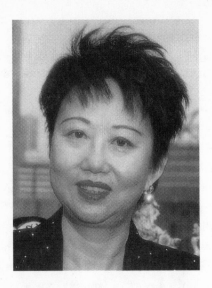

Jannie Tay, PhD (Hons.) is the Managing Director of The Hour Glass Limited, a listed company in Singapore. It is a leading wholesaler and retailer of high-quality, distinctive timepieces and jewellery in the Asia Pacific, which she and her husband co-founded in 1979. In 1995, she started Oyster Cove development, a 400-acre residential/hotel resort development in Gold Coast, Queensland, Australia. She is the President of both ASEAN Business Forum and Singapore Retailers Association and is the first woman to attain these positions. Jannie is also the founding President of Women For Women Association and the immediate past President of the International Women's Forum. In October 2000, she was invited to join a group of global business leaders to form the inaugural Business Advisory Council for The United Nations Office for Project Services (UNOPS). A recipient of many awards, she was honoured as one of fifty Leading Women Entrepreneurs of the World in 1997 and is a tireless worker for numerous charitable, family and women's causes.

Jannie Tay

For me, menopause was simply a time in my life when my period stopped and that's it – all normal, really.

I'm happy I don't have a period. I work very hard, often spend six or eight months of the year out of the country. To tell you the truth, even though I've been through it, I wouldn't even know what menopause was all about. There was never any discussion about menopause among my friends. Why should there be? There's no need to make a big issue of it. A lot of people I knew had dropped their babies before I even knew they were pregnant. I think our need to discuss and analyse menopause is a psychological pressure, a seed planted in our head. I think we need to avoid the pressure.

Apart from a few, minor hot flushes I had absolutely no symptoms during menopause. I just lead a very normal life with no medication, nothing. A lot of people tell me I'm wrong not to take anything, but I had a check-up last year and everything's fine. The doctor didn't even ask me about menopause.

Maybe the changes in hormones are critical to some people, but they haven't been an issue for me. I haven't been sick for three years except for a very mild cold. We are constantly reminded to question our health. We say, 'My doctor tells me to do this,' or 'I should be feeling like that.' If I feel drained or unwell, I might sit by the beach to recuperate, but the first thing that many of us seem to do is run to the doctor. Why do you think that is?

Maybe it's the psychology of women to accept things as they come rather than to challenge them. Then again, it could have something to do with cultural background. I think most Australian women have an expectation that certain things will start happening when they reach menopause because that's the norm.

But in Asia we practically don't even know what it is. None of us ever discussed it. Okay, we know when we are reaching menopause because our period doesn't come, and we probably need to be careful with our bones, but that's about it. Most working women are so busy with their lives that they have no time to think about themselves. It's the suggestions that we put in people's minds about changes in their lives and changes in their relationships that make it difficult.

If someone hadn't told me that the hot flushes meant menopause, I wouldn't have even made a connection. I've flown through it, really. And the only distinctive thing is that I didn't have my period for over a year, and then it came back again briefly and, from then on, nothing. So I've gone through menopause without even realising it.

I've been in business now for eighteen years. If I compare myself to what I was like when I first started in business, I'd have to say that I'm much calmer now. I'm not stressed and I'm not as excited about things. I have this balance where I know my strengths and weaknesses, what my challenges are. I don't respond with negativity, I just walk away from it. I'm very calm about most things because I know it is not me, it is others' perception or judgement of me but it is not important to me.

I don't get angry very much now. When you learn to understand life and situations there is nothing to get angry about. Very rarely do I find myself at the angry stage. If I do it's always a response to other people's unfair actions, but even that I have learnt to let go. You cannot change someone's perceptions and judgements. Just let it be.

I think I'm in a more spiritual and balanced, serene mode. I don't get hassled or troubled. I accept challenges as they come and I respond to what has to be done positively, with positive goals in mind.

I sleep well at night. Whether I go to bed early or late, I sleep the whole night through. With a mental constitution like mine I can get on a plane and I'm asleep within five minutes. When I arrive at my destination, whether it's three hours or half a day or a day later, I wake up and there I am. So the ability to sleep and catch a nap is great for me.

I don't ever think of my life in terms of achievement. I think of what I am passionate about and enjoy doing, and as long as I love doing something then I am achieving. I do what I do because I believe it's my purpose in life. I was told my main purpose in life was to build a bridge between east and west, to make networks between women and men, so I look at the challenges associated with those and manage them as I need to at the time.

I'm beginning to flow with this purpose and to sense intuitively and recognise that it is a strong part of my life now. What's really important is your attitude and to sort out what life means to you, its purpose. I've accepted the responsibility of my life's purpose and the challenges that I will face in pursuing this. I will work towards it with God and his spirit guiding me.

Perhaps because I was never really ambitious, I never set myself goals in terms of business and finance. I know I can be successful if I do my best in everything I do and am passionate about it. In business, my family supports me. I grow as a person. If life is just about business or money, then I don't think I would want to do it. And if it was just a job then I wouldn't want to do it either. I think I grow as a person because I enjoy what I do. I'm passionate about it.

When I was fifty, I started evaluating my life, mainly because until then I had focused on building the business for my kids and looking after their needs. Then suddenly I thought, Hang on, why am I working all my life for my kids and dream of them being someone when they may not want to be?

In a way, I built the business for my kids because I wanted them to have a better future. I loved my work, but I wanted them to have something too. That became part of my purpose in life at the earlier stage.

But then I looked back and thought, Okay, if the kids don't really want it, fine. I think I'll sell out, take it easy and enjoy myself.

I decided that now my kids have a life of their own, I'd better have a life of my own too. And the moment I started thinking of a life of my own, I knew what I wanted to do. I really wanted to meditate. I wanted to write, paint and dance. I don't think I would want to do any more business if it wasn't such a huge part of my life on so many levels.

So the bottom line is as long as we love and are passionate about what we are doing we grow with it, and we enjoy it, because it's a learning experience. It helps you grow spiritually, mentally and physically, and eternally.

Chapter Eleven
Exercise – why do it?

Why do it? How exercise prevents loss of muscle and bone mass. The benefits of weight-bearing exercise: strength training, walking, aerobic exercise. How to check your heart and pulse rates. Other cardiovascular activities. The benefits of exercise, including prevention of heart disease and increase in bone mass. Studies into the combined effects of hormone replacement therapy and exercise. What form of exercise to choose. A warning about the dangers of over-exercising.

Regular exercise is extremely important for fitness. It also helps us to stay relaxed, to sleep and feel better, and helps to reduce the symptoms of menopause.

After exercise you feel fantastic, so make it part of your daily routine. Exercise ensures permanent weight management, gives you more energy and prevents osteoporosis, diabetes and heart disease. In a nutshell, exercise increases the quality of life.

Nature has made exercise accessible to us. It can cost nothing, there are no chemicals involved, and it is not difficult to do. Often, our greatest barrier to establishing a regular exercise routine is motivation.

By the age of forty, women begin to lose bone. This loss increases as they age and accelerates for five to seven years after menopause, when their oestrogen concentration is low. By the time women reach sixty-five, they have lost an average of 25 to 35 per cent of their total bone mass.

Exercise helps prevent bone loss, improves muscle mass, strength and body balance. Maintaining strong bones is important for the prevention of osteoporosis and related bone fractures. Increasing bone mass by up to 3 to 5 per cent reduces the risk of fracture by 20 to 30 per cent.

Women begin to lose muscle mass around the time of menopause, resulting in a loss of body strength and a general lack of vigour. Our bodies have over 600 muscles responsible for movement that account for over a third of our total body weight. As we age, we lose muscle and gain fat in a process known as 'sarcoperia'. From the age of forty, women usually lose close to 200 grams of muscle each year and replace it with an equal amount of fat. As women age, and especially if they are not physically active, this condition worsens. By the age of eighty, women may have lost about a third of their muscle mass. A sensible eating program and regular exercise are the most effective remedies for controlling weight gain in mid-life.

As we age, we are less physically active than when we were younger. The decline in muscle mass from less activity slows down our metabolism, the process that turns what we eat into energy or stores it as fat.

Most of our bone calcium is laid down in our early teens. It increases as we grow, peaks by the age of twenty, then levels out, and finally begins to decline by the time we are forty. Most bone loss occurs within three to five years after menopause and continues at a rate of 1 per cent each year. At this stage in life, it is important to prevent bone loss. Changes to your life, such as regular exercise, can achieve this.

Preserving bone density and improving muscle mass and balance reduces the incidence of falls, thus reducing bone fractures. Fractures associated with low bone mass are increasing at an alarming rate. About half of all women above the age of fifty will suffer from osteoporotic fractures.

To reap the full benefit of exercise, it must be regular. Women who have undertaken weight-bearing exercise such as aerobics, tennis, resistance exercise or jogging since early adulthood can increase their bone mass and density before menopause sets in.

Although weight-bearing exercise is most beneficial if started earlier, women who begin exercising at menopause can restore 3 to 4 per cent of their bone mass yearly and will maintain this level as long as they continue physical activity.

If exercise stops, bone loss will continue as before, and women who drop their exercise routines altogether will return to the bone-loss levels of more sedentary women within several years.

Regular exercise has a significant effect on body composition in older women.

Weight-bearing exercises and strength and resistance training all help in maintaining bone density and preventing osteoporosis. Weight-bearing exercises use our large muscles and ensure that the body supports its own weight while exercising. This type of exercise is excellent for maintaining bone strength.

> 'My mother told me not to worry about anything during menopause. She said that a lot of women go on about it, but in reality it's very little trouble. Her advice must have worked. I suppose I have her strong genes to thank for that.'
>
> SHEILA SCOTTER

Weight-bearing exercises, such as jogging, walking, aerobics classes, tennis, volleyball, netball, badminton and stair-climbing, increase bone density more than non weight-bearing exercises, such as cycling and swimming. Weight-bearing exercise is known to preserve bone density and has positive effects on risk factors for osteoporotic fractures while the strong aerobic component of this type of exercise prevents age-related accumulation of abdominal fat in older men and women.

This view is supported by recent research. One study looks at how different exercise programs affect bone-mineral density (Kohrt *et al.*, 1997). Women, aged sixty to seventy-four, were given a set of exercises that introduced skeletal stress through ground-reaction force, such as walking or jogging, and another set of exercises that introduced skeletal stress through joint-reaction force, such as weight-lifting and rowing.

The two programs resulted in significant and similar increases in bone-mineral density of the whole body when compared to a non-exercise control group. The control group showed no significant changes in bone mineral density.

There are several types of weight-bearing exercises favoured by clinicians, dieticians and physiotherapists because they are simple, cheap and provide great health benefits and protection against heart disease and osteoporosis. These include strength training, walking and aerobic exercises.

'When my doctor examined me he said, "Do you do any exercise?" And I said, "The only exercise I do is looking around for the nearest couch to sit down on."'

JEANNE PRATT

Strength training is an important form of exercise for older women. It is a mode of exercise in which the muscles work against a resistance sufficiently high to increase strength. This was shown in a study published in the *Journal of the American Medical Association* (Nelson, 1994).

Strength training increases muscle mass and strength and might be effective in preventing osteoporosis. Strength-training exercise delays and often reverses the sarcopenia process for decades, decreases the risk of heart disease, relieves arthritis symptoms, improves metabolism and boosts overall body spirit.

Nelson found that women can gain enormous health benefits from simple strengthening exercises. After a year of twice-weekly strength training, forty postmenopausal women aged between fifty and seventy had regained bone mass and increased muscle strength when compared to women in the same age-range who undertook no exercise.

Within two months of the study, participants had doubled the weight they could lift and steadily improved throughout the year. The women became leaner and trimmer, and maintained their overall body weight without any change to their eating habits. They replaced body fat with muscle and lost centimetres around their waist and hips. Participants also showed improvement in body balance and flexibility, were almost 30 per cent more active and, after the program, had bodies up to twenty years more youthful.

In her book, *Strong Women Stay Young* (1997), Nelson has designed a practical, home-based, strength-training program that fits easily into the daily routine. It is suggested that the forty-minute program, consisting of eight simple exercises done in standing or sitting positions, should be performed at least twice weekly. Nelson's preliminary data show a significant improvement in body strength after just four weeks on the program. In her subsequent book, *Strong Women, Strong Bones* (2000), Nelson focuses on an exercise program that includes strengthening work designed to promote bone health and prevent osteoporosis.

Undertaking a home-based, strength-training program requires a few inexpensive items, including dumb bells, ankle weights, a sturdy chair, a floor mat, comfortable clothes and properly fitted shoes. Once you have these items, all it takes is motivation and a positive attitude to start, and maintain, your own exercise program.

Kashiwa and Rippe in their book *Fitness Walking for Women* (1987) outline a low-impact exercise program for women of all ages and in all different situations that helps with weight gain, stiff muscles and joints, tension, heart trouble and loss of bone and muscle mass.

Studies published in this area show that exercise, either alone or combined with a healthy-eating program, significantly reduces body fat and leads to weight loss.

Most of the weight lost from dieting without an exercise program is muscle rather than fat. Walking is a weight-bearing exercise that burns fat, controls your appetite, expends more calories and increases muscle mass. Walking has no special requirements other than a personal commitment to ensuring a three to four times a week program of about thirty to forty minutes for every walking session.

Aerobic activity is exceptionally good for strengthening the heart as it provides cardiovascular training. Aerobic activities include jogging, cycling or aerobics classes. Aerobic exercise elevates our pulse and heart rates and is most beneficial when the heart rate is increased to a target range of 60 to 70 per cent of our maximum aerobic capacity. Pulse rate is a good gauge of the intensity of an exercise, and you should aim to maintain an elevated pulse rate for up to ten minutes before easing back and cooling off.

The easiest way to calculate your maximum pulse rate is to subtract your age from 220 and then multiply the result by 0.7. If you are fifty-six, for example, your heart rate would be calculated at 115 beats a minute. This is the number of beats a minute when you are exercising at 70 per cent of your maximum heart rate.

To check that you are exercising in your optimum heart-rate zone, exercise for ten to fifteen minutes and then feel for your pulse at your neck or wrist. Count your pulse beats for thirty seconds and double this figure for your exercising heart rate. You may also wish to buy an inexpensive heart-rate monitor to check your pulse.

Cardiovascular endurance, or aerobic activity, is an extremely important element of fitness. Cardiovascular activity helps control blood pressure, blood sugar, body weight and levels of beneficial cholesterol, improves self-esteem and reduces anxiety.

Outdoor aerobic activities such as walking, jogging, rowing, cycling and skiing are one way of obtaining the benefits of cardiovascular endurance, but you can achieve the same results with indoor aerobic exercises or resistance training. Using machines like exercise bikes, treadmills and rowing machines is one way. Alternatively, an aerobic exercise like dancing is fun, sociable and keeps you moving.

Lower impact exercises such as yoga or swimming can also be incorporated into a regular exercise routine.

Yoga helps to relax the body and the mind, restores your energy levels, increases overall flexibility and provides an incredible feeling of well-being. When combined with a weight-bearing exercise program, it contributes to an all-round improvement in health.

Swimming can be a valuable cardiovascular activity that improves circulation, tones muscles, relieves stress and improves sleep. Water is refreshing and provides less impact on your joints.

Warming up and cooling down with five to ten minutes of slow, steady stretching should be part of every exercise program. Stretches should be gradual and relaxed. After-exercise stretching prevents muscles from tightening up. Stretching helps reduce anxiety and muscle tension, and lowers blood pressure and your breathing rate.

Whether you are exercising alone at home, walking, playing tennis with a friend, or participating in an aerobics class, maintain your program and your enthusiasm by setting realistic goals. Many forms of exercise use almost all of our 200-odd bones and 600-odd muscles, and the health benefits to the body are enormous. There is no need to make exercise a chore. You can achieve sufficient health benefits through a moderate, achievable and enjoyable exercise routine.

Fifty per cent of postmenopausal women do not follow any exercise program. Don't become part of this statistic. Start by simply going for a walk, or, if the weather is bad, doing some stretching exercises on the floor. Most importantly, have fun and enjoy your exercise.

Postmenopausal women who exercise have an improved sense of well-being, high self-esteem and self-image, and are happy. This may be because during exercise the adrenal glands release the hormone noradrenaline, a hormone associated with a positive attitude.

Women who exercise have fewer symptoms of menopause, such as hot flushes, and greater cardio-respiratory capacity than women who do not exercise. Incremental exercise increases aerobic fitness in women who are one to three years postmenopause. Regular exercise helps women lose fat and control body weight, and it provides better appetite control and better long-term weight management.

Exercise stimulates the parts of the nervous system responsible for controlling 'stress hormones' and reduces the levels of these chemicals in the body, inducing feelings of calm. It enhances your long-term ability to deal with stress, anxiety and, possibly, depression, and it improves sleep.

Exercise in older people increases the oxygen concentration supplied to the brain, improving mental agility, concentration, and the speed at which data and information are processed. Exercise stimulates the immune system and, as a result, can lower death rates from all possible causes.

Exercising slows down the loss of dopamine, a neurotransmitter in the brain that prevents symptoms of shaking that come with old age and in Parkinson's disease. Exercise improves your metabolism by normalising blood sugar and stimulating the uptake of sugar by the muscle tissue. This has the great benefit of lowering the risk of diabetes.

One of the better documented benefits of regular exercise is its effect of reducing cardiovascular disease. Other studies show that exercising for just three months is enough to significantly decrease blood pressure, total cholesterol, triglycerides and low-density (bad cholesterol) lipoproteins and increase high-density (beneficial cholesterol) lipoproteins and physical fitness. HDL appears to have some protective effect of lowering coronary artery disease.

Heart disease is the primary killer of men and women, and cardiovascular diseases account for 50 per cent of all deaths. Aerobic exercise, power walking and strength-training exercises improve the strength and efficiency of the cardiac muscle, reduce blood pressure, increase blood-flow to every cell in the body and may be effective in decreasing the occurrence of coronary artery disease that leads to angina and heart attacks.

Given the enormous benefits of exercise, it is no surprise that sedentary women are more likely to suffer from heart attacks than women who exercise regularly. Research indicates that, although hardening of the arteries is related to age, the magnitude of its occurrence could be reduced with regular exercise.

A Melbourne-based study by Cameron and Dart (1994) found that the main function of the arteries, known as 'arterial compliance', is played out in the control of cardiovascular disease. Arterial compliance is related to the elasticity of an artery and its ability to respond appropriately to increased blood volume. Exercise increases arterial compliance, possibly through altered lipid and lipoprotein metabolism, and helps the arteries adapt better to changes in blood volume.

The specific type, intensity and frequency of exercise needed to produce the optimal increase in arterial compliance and a reduced risk in cardiovascular disease varies for each individual. To make the most of cardiac health benefits, however, exercise must be consistent and lifelong.

Physically active women have less uterine and ovarian cancer than sedentary women. This is also true for the incidence of breast cancer in physically active, perimenopausal women. Exercise lengthens the menstrual cycle and decreases the concentration of the oestrogen and progesterone that acts on the breast cells.

Regular exercise in the perimenopausal years reduces the overall exposure to oestrogen enormously, providing additional benefits to women in this age group. Reduced exposure to oestrogen might explain why women who exercise get fewer hot flushes than sedentary women.

'I have a trainer for motivation and for help with my exercises, and he is absolutely fabulous. He's also a physiotherapist and a fitness fanatic. He pushes me to the limit, and then I go over the limit with him.'

LILLIAN FRANK

Exercise also increases bone mass by providing a mechanical stimulus on the bone which, in turn, promotes bone growth and formation. This is demonstrated in physical deprivation studies, where the effects of immobilisation and weightlessness, similar to those experienced during space travel, decrease bone mass density more readily than the effects of oestrogen or calcium deprivation. Total inactivity, such as confinement to bed, causes the bones to lose calcium, making them more brittle.

In contrast, moderate weight-bearing exercise may delay vertebrate bone loss in postmenopausal women. Smith and Gilligan (1991) studied three groups of women at the mean age of eighty for three years. One group sat in a chair and exercised their arms and legs three times a week for thirty minutes, another group supplemented their exercise program with calcium and the third control group did not exercise or take supplements. Each participant's bone calcification was measured at the beginning and the end of the study. The authors found that the first group of women gained the most calcium, and that the third group lost bone calcium.

Exercise strengthens bones by stabilising them and improving bone density, strengthens ligaments, cartilage and tendons, improves balance and flexibility, and decreases the risk of falling and fracturing bones.

Exercise and hormone replacement therapy on their own stabilise or increase bone density. This improvement might reduce the risk of bone fracture. However, the combination of exercise and hormone replacement therapy has given conflicting results.

In our own laboratory at Victoria University, we investigated hormone replacement therapy and walking, independently and in combination, to determine which treatment regime provided most benefits to bone loss in postmenopausal women (Honisett *et al.*, 2001).

'I've noticed lately that I'm nowhere near the agile tennis player I used to be. Nowadays, I'm relying heavily on cunning at the net and a hard serve.'

ELAINE CANTY

When postmenopausal women were placed on a twelve-week program combining hormone replacement therapy (transdermal oestrogen patches and daily progesterone tablets) or a placebo and incremental walking exercises, following eight weeks of hormone replacement therapy or placebo alone, we found that hormone replacement significantly reduces bone resorption. A combined treatment, incorporating walking and hormone replacement therapy provided no added benefits in comparison to hormonal therapy alone.

So far there has been little research into the combined effects of hormone replacement therapy and exercise on cardiovascular parameters. A Melbourne-based study by Waddell *et al.*, 1999 found that, after six weeks of hormone replacement therapy, arterial compliance improved in postmenopausal women. When these women were taken off the hormonal therapy, after four weeks their arterial compliance decreased, and improved again when the program was resumed.

One study (Lindheim *et al.*, 1994) assesses how moderate exercise programs, with and without oral oestrogen replacement, affect the levels of lipids and lipoproteins in postmenopausal women. This study found that oestrogen therapy alone and exercise alone had the greatest beneficial effect on lipids by significantly decreasing total cholesterol levels and the low-density lipoprotein (LDL) cholesterol, and significantly increasing the high-density (HDL) cholesterol. The combined hormone replacement therapy and exercise program, however, did not demonstrate added improvements in lipid parameters.

Other studies published in this area (Prince *et al.*, 1991 and Heikkinen *et al.*, 1991) studied the independent and combined effects of exercise and hormone replacement therapy on bone mineral density. These studies reported conflicting results in the use of a combined regimen in postmenopausal women.

With such limited evidence, it is difficult to speculate conclusively on the effects of hormone replacement therapy and exercise. More studies are needed.

Overall, we can say that exercise and hormone replacement therapy may be effective in preventing osteoporosis by increasing and maintaining bone mass, but further work in this area is also required to substantiate the exact exercising regimes that produce the most beneficial results.

How much exercise is effective for maintaining total health but moderate enough to incorporate into most people's lives? There are plenty of books, audio and videotapes that offer effective exercise programs. The best program to prevent osteoporosis is one that combines different types of exercise: weight-bearing, weight and strength-training. A combined walking and strength-training program, for example, is an exercise regime that can provide most benefits. Swimming and cycling may be of great value in improving respiratory and cardiovascular fitness but, because they are non weight-bearing exercises, they do not prevent bone loss.

The choice of exercise must reflect your way of life to be enjoyable. Choose a type of exercise that also suits your personality and social needs. Sports like tennis, netball or badminton can offer great social benefits and encourage a regular exercise pattern. Whatever exercise you choose, you will need comfortable attire and lots of motivation and good will. For postmenopausal women, the program of choice should be of thirty to forty minutes duration and undertaken three to four times a week.

A regular exercise program should be a high priority for every postmenopausal woman. To be effective and prevent bone loss, it must be part of the daily routine.

'As far as exercise goes, I used to be the absolute couch potato. It was only four years ago that I found a little gym that was very near where I lived. Gradually I have got to really enjoy it. Now I go three times a week.'

STEPHANIE ALEXANDER

Other habits, such as alcohol consumption, cigarette smoking and excessive caffeine intake, have a negative effect on bones, particularly in women. Excessive intake of alcohol lowers bone mass and can lead to osteoporosis. Nicotine from tobacco smoking can lower the blood's oestrogen production, thus reducing bone strength. And excessive caffeine intake may disrupt the way calcium is absorbed in the body.

Adding milk, which is readily absorbed into the bloodstream, to coffee can counterbalance the negative impact of caffeine. Although the social aspects of a chat over a cup of coffee can be very relaxing and even therapeutic, we need to be mindful of ensuring moderation for a well-balanced and healthy life.

Moderation is a very important consideration. A very small number of women can become physiologically addicted to exercise. Going to extremes in exercise can be just as detrimental to your life as excessive caffeine or alcohol intake. Over-exercising can lower your immune system, making it more susceptible to colds, flu and injuries, and can cause various psychological problems such as mood swings or even depression. Extreme, strenuous exercise in young athletes can lead to irregular menstruation, or periods that stop altogether, and can lower bone density.

When combined, hormone replacement therapy and exercise may increase bone mass and minimise the effects of osteoporosis but, so far, limited data are available on the effects of these therapies on cardiovascular disease.

The needs and wishes of postmenopausal women should be considered along with their medical history and relevant scientific data, to help them make an informed choice about an appropriate management method that will maintain compliance and provide greatest benefit.

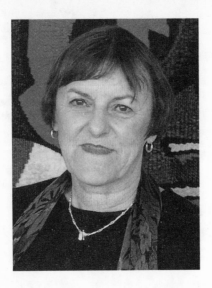

Sue Walker is a graduate of Melbourne University, where she is now engaged in post-graduate studies. A long-standing involvement with the visual and decorative arts, initially in education, and an interest in architecture inspired by her father, led to her appointment in 1976 as the founding Director of the Victorian Tapestry Workshop. In this position she has played a key role in bringing the art of tapestry into the mainstream of Australia's cultural life. She has been responsible for initiating opportunities and collaborations for more than 300 artists from Australia and overseas to work in tapestry and for the placing of tapestries in many significant public locations. As Director of the Workshop she has curated and toured numerous travelling exhibitions to major international centres throughout the world. In 1988 she convened an International Tapestry Symposium in Melbourne. She has edited and published several full-colour catalogues and lectured at numerous study days and conferences in many world centres.

Sue Walker

I had a hysterectomy when I was fifty, so my experience of menopause is probably a little different from most women. Of course, I had menopausal symptoms before then, but, to tell you the truth, there were so many things going on in my life at the time that it's difficult to untangle it all. It was a very torrid period through those years.

I suppose my symptoms had already started before the hysterectomy. I remember the hot flush stuff, a sense of heat, that kind of thing. And I remember I used to burst into tears rather unexpectedly. But my emotional state was probably mixed up with my mother's death, my children leaving home, problems with my marriage and worries about my own health. It was all quite a mess.

Around this time it was recommended that I have a hysterectomy because I had fibroids. These days you probably wouldn't have needed such invasive surgery for something like fibroids, but back then a hysterectomy was the recommended action. On the advice of my doctor I asked the surgeon to keep one of my ovaries, but I was plunged into a type of menopause as a result of the hysterectomy.

I used hormone replacement therapy to control the menopausal symptoms and have remained on it ever since. My doctor has recommended that I keep taking it to help with other possible problems like asthma, cardiovascular disease and Alzheimer's disease as I get older.

One symptom that did alarm me at the time was the migraines. I found out much later that migraines are actually a very common symptom of the menopause, but I had never experienced them before and I was quite alarmed at first. I actually had some tests to try and work out what was going on, but the doctors didn't seem to know why I was getting them. It was only afterwards when I talked with other women that I found out how common migraines actually were.

The first of these migraines was just around the time my mother died. It was a stressful time and I was very tense. I remember driving up a hill in Canberra when I saw these flickering lights in front of my eyes. I was really tired and quite stressed.

Watching while Mum slowly deteriorated with cancer and juggling my work around spending time with her and making sure Dad was okay too was quite a struggle. I remember vividly the day a friend said to me that now I needed to take the lead and be the one who made the decisions. Suddenly roles were reversed. It was quite a revelation. While our parents are alive, we often tend to see ourselves as still children. It felt strange in a position where I was now the adult decision-maker.

I'd often rush off from work to be with Mum and give Dad a break from his demanding role as caregiver. This went on for more than a year. It was a pretty rough time for all of us.

After Mum's death, I spent much more time with my father – we supported each other really. It was quite good that I was free to do that, and I remember that period as a special time for both of us. He lived for another ten years.

I didn't really look for a lot of support from my family and friends during that time but was pleased when it was offered. It sometimes seemed I was always the one doing the supporting. Even my daughter was going through a difficult period.

I usually had quite a lot of men friends, but not as many women friends. Of course, for part of the time my husband was around to provide some support, but it might have been helpful if I had found time to talk about the things I was going through with some-one else.

Looking back, it resulted in an enormous period of introspection and growth. In fact, it cemented my desire to return to do some Fine Arts study at Melbourne University. I've been studying ever since, and am now studying for a Ph.D in Fine Arts. I've made some great friends at university, and I've continued to some extent to be involved in the department.

I've continued to do my job as Director of the Tapestry Workshop and managed to maintain my studies as well. In a way, the studying took the place of some of my family relationships. I did quite a lot of work then, and I've managed to get through a Masters Prelim degree as well as completing some terrific special studies. I loved it, and I still love it. I can see lots of connections between my writing, my work and my study.

I feel that I have gained a lot through the experiences I have lived through over the past ten years. How much menopause has played a part, I don't really know. I think that those difficult personal experiences, and the relationships that followed on from them, have really taught me a lot about myself.

I've got a really lovely relationship now, which makes me feel extremely lucky and firm in the knowledge that there isn't really anything in my life that I couldn't cope with now. In the past, when change has seemed inevitable, I often felt I would never be able to cope. Now anything seems possible. I love being in my mid-sixties. I absolutely love it. I love being a grandmother and find enormous pleasure in my three granddaughters. I don't feel at all like I'm sixty-four. I have a great friend who is ninety-two, and she doesn't feel ninety-two either.

You learn to take less notice of the changes now. You simply accommodate them. I used to hate it when my eyesight was changing, and I'd continually have to put my glasses on and off and back on again. Now I'm used to it. I have a pair of graduated lenses that I can wear all the time. And it's like that with most things. I just look for ways to make things that little bit easier.

I don't have much of a plan for the future, except that I'd like to keep healthy, and maintain close involvement with my children and their families. I also want to be sure that I don't stay on at the Tapestry Workshop to the point where the place is suffering as a result, so I'm talking to the Board about succession planning and that sort of thing.

I think that there are some interesting business models and if the right person came along to be a successor, I could start planning to wind down. I would like to travel more, but I haven't quite got to the point yet where I can say, 'Let's go to France for a month.' I'm still too focused on my work.

I've always been fairly active. I love swimming and I try to swim about three days a week. I've been playing golf and I love walking, but I don't think I've consciously developed my fitness regime – it just sort of happened that way.

I've always eaten a fairly healthy diet. I don't eat much sugar, and I don't drink much. I don't eat as much meat as I did in the past, but, other than that, I can't say that I've made any great changes to my diet.

As far as security for my future goes, I think that there is always an underlying concern and a responsibility, especially when you have a family to worry about. I suppose my brother and I feel a bit more financially secure because of the backing from our father's estate. I didn't really manage to start putting much into my superannuation until about a few years ago, so this wouldn't really have kept me going for very long. Just that bit extra from Dad's estate has helped a lot. It's nice to be able to feel some security for the future.

Chapter Twelve
Food for thought

The importance of sensible eating and maintaining normal body weight. What is a healthy diet? The different elements in food – their role in our nutrition and which foods contain them. What kind of diet women in midlife should have – and what to avoid eating.

Being healthy is more than just being free of disease, it also means feeling good about yourself, being contented and being in control of your life. Menopause is a time to assess your way of living and how it might be affecting your health.

To experience total health, you may need to make a few changes by eating a well-balanced diet, getting regular exercise and reducing and controlling stress.

A sensible eating program is important throughout life. As you get older your nutritional requirements change, your metabolism slows down, your body absorbs fewer nutrients and you require fewer calories. You may even exercise less. If you continue to eat the same amount and types of food as before, you will probably put on weight. It is very important to guard against weight gain as this can increase your risk of heart disease, which will already be increased by your diminishing levels of oestrogen.

It is important to manage what and how much you eat and how you keep your body in shape. For many women, weight has never been a problem. For others, life has been a constant battle with a multitude of diets. Weight gain results when the amount of calories you consume exceeds the amount of calories you use through metabolic and physical activities.

Most women notice an increase in weight at this transitional stage in their lives. This weight might be evenly distributed throughout the body or it will begin to appear as extra bulk around the midriff.

Carrying just a few extra kilograms at mid-life can be an advantage as your body can convert some of this fat into oestrogen when needed, helping to diminish the effects of low oestrogen levels. Obesity, however, is a health risk. When you carry extra kilograms your heart and lungs have to work hard. Overweight women are more likely to develop diabetes and cardiovascular disease, and the extra load places enormous strain on backs and joints.

As you approach menopause, it becomes very important to remain within a normal weight range. If your weight has been fluctuating as a result of fad diets, now is the time to develop an eating pattern that is healthy and that you can follow for the rest of your life.

Diet is important at any time of life, but when you reach forty it is really important to watch what you eat. The perimenopausal and menopausal years require special dietary needs which, when met, can help you have an easy passage through menopause and reduce the likelihood of associated postmenopausal health problems such as cardiovascular diseases, osteoporosis and even breast cancer.

The most appropriate diet for women approaching mid-life is one that is high in whole grains, vegetables, fruit and dairy products. If you decide to reduce the amount of food you consume, either to control weight or to suppress your appetite, you must maintain a well-rounded nutrient intake. This should come from a variety of foods which will give you the highest number of nutrients for the number of calories you consume.

The healthy diet pyramid divides food groups into three basic categories: foods to eat in small amounts, foods to eat moderately and foods to eat most. Foods to eat in plentiful amounts sit at base of the pyramid and include breads (wholegrain and wholemeal), cereals, pasta, rice, vegetables and fruit. Foods you should eat moderately sit in the middle third of the pyramid and include milk, low-fat cheese, yogurt, lean meats, poultry, fish, nuts and eggs. Foods at the top of the pyramid are those most likely to cause weight gain and heart disease and should be eaten in small quantities. These include sugars, butter, margarine, salt, creams and alcohol.

It is important to eat low-fat foods more often and to choose a variety of foods from each group to eat daily.

A nutrient is a substance in food that the body uses to promote normal growth, maintenance and repair. The major nutrients are carbohydrates, lipids (fats) and proteins. Nutrients required in smaller amounts are vitamins and minerals. One further category, water, is not a nutrient in the strict sense but it accounts for 60 per cent of the volume of food we eat. For this reason, it is considered a major nutrient.

Most foods offer a combination of nutrients, so it is important to manage your diet to ensure that you are eating foods that supply sufficient amounts of the nutrients that your body needs.

There are three types of carbohydrates: simple or monosaccharide, disaccharide, and polysaccharide or complex. Glucose or blood sugar is a simple carbohydrate. It is the final molecule in the process of carbohydrate breakdown and is used to fuel the body. Some tissues, such as brain cells and red blood cells, use glucose as their major source of energy. Another simple carbohydrate is fructose found in fruit and young vegetables. Simple carbohydrates are also found in carbonated drinks and ice creams.

Disaccharides consist of sucrose, found in cane sugar, fruits and vege-tables; lactose, found in milk; and maltose, found in germinating seeds.

Polysaccharides include starches, fibre and glycogen, a storage form of carbohydrate in humans and animals.

Complex carbohydrates provide the body with vital energy and include breads, cereals, rice, pasta, potatoes and nuts. A healthy diet should include 125 to 175 grams of complex carbohydrates each day, or 55 to 60 per cent of your total daily calorie intake.

Fibres are either soluble or insoluble. The soluble fibres (oatmeal, legumes, bananas, apples, carrots and corn) tend to form a gel when they are in contact with water. About a third of the total fibre in a typical diet is soluble. Insoluble fibre or 'roughage' (whole grain, wheat bran, mature fruits and vegetables such as cabbage, green peppers and broccoli) remains almost intact as it passes through the entire gut. This important fibre keeps the gut healthy, promotes regular bowel movement and reduces the risk of heart disease and breast cancer. The recommended daily intake of fibre is 25 grams a day.

'Ultimately, I do believe you can have it all. You can have a fabulous career, and you can have children. I had my first child in my early twenties and the last one when I was thirty-three. There's nothing I regret about any of it.'

JAN WADE

The lipids include saturated fats, monosaturated fats and polyunsaturated fats and are derived from plant and animal sources. Lipids help the body to absorb fat-soluble vitamins (A, E and D), provide a cushioning layer for the body's internal organs, help to insulate the skin and are a major energy source for the muscles.

Saturated fats tend to be solid at room temperature and include animal-derived foods, such as cheese, eggs, lard, butter, meat and milk, and plant-derived foods such as coconut and palm oils.

Monosaturated fats stay liquid or soft at room temperature and are found in fish, olive and peanut oils, peanut butter and avocado.

Polyunsaturated fats also remain liquid or soft at room temperature and are found in almonds, walnuts, corn, sunflower and sesame oils and soft margarine.

Lean chicken, beef and pork contain a mixture of all three types of fat, mostly monounsaturated.

Twenty-five to 30 per cent of your total daily calorie intake should include lipids, but you should keep your consumption of saturated fats to below 10 per cent of the total fats you eat. Postmenopausal women should limit their daily fat consumption to below 20 per cent of their total calorie intake to maintain a normal body weight.

The two types of proteins are complete proteins, including eggs, milk, fish, poultry, beef and lamb, and incomplete proteins such as legumes, soybean, lentils, vegetables, nuts and seeds. Proteins are the basic building-blocks of life and, next to water, are the most powerful substances in our bodies, making up 18 to 20 per cent of our total body weight. Proteins build and repair muscle and body tissues and support our cells, skin, hair, muscle, blood vessels and internal organs. We need to eat at least 60 grams of protein every day.

The vitamins we eat are either fat soluble (vitamins A, D, E and K) or water soluble (vitamins B and C). Fat-soluble vitamins are found in green vegetables and many of the large food groups. Water-soluble vitamins are derived from foods such as fruits, vegetables, lean meats, legumes, eggs and fish.

Although vitamins are not part of the body's basic building-blocks, or used as energy sources, they are needed in small amounts for growth and good health. Each vitamin has a recommended daily dosage and these are discussed in the chapter on supplements.

Minerals are found in dairy products and meat. There are seven minerals in dairy foods – calcium, phosphorus, sulfur, sodium, chloride, magnesium and potassium. Meat contains trace minerals including iron, iodine, zinc, copper, fluorine, selenium, chromium, manganese and cobalt. Minerals are not part of the body's energy source, but they do work with other nutrients to contribute to our body functions. Minerals and their recommended daily intake are also discussed in the chapter on supplements.

A practical diet for women in menopause should aim to reduce short-term symptoms of menopause such as hot flushes, night sweats, anxiety, insomnia, weight gain and fatigue, and to minimise the occurrence of postmenopausal health conditions such as an increased risk of cardiovascular disease, breast cancer or osteoporosis.

Women in menopause need to increase the amount of complex carbohydrates they eat while reducing their fat intake. The starch in complex carbohydrates provides a ready source of energy and regulates our blood-sugar levels without promoting weight gain. We can increase our complex carbohydrate intake by eating more fruit, vegetables, cereals, breads, pasta and rice, and by eating more high-fibre foods such as brown rice, wholemeal pasta and breads.

Aim to reduce the amount of simple carbohydrates and sugar in your diet. Processed carbohydrates and simple sugars put on weight, increase blood-sugar levels and lethargy, increase the amount of calcium our bodies excrete and set up an imbalance in the ratio of HDL to LDL cholesterols. HDL cholesterol is beneficial to the body, but LDL cholesterol is quite harmful and should be kept within its normal levels.

Fats also need careful monitoring. Try to increase the amount of monounsaturated fats you eat and avoid foods high in polyunsaturated and saturated fats. Use olive oil for cooking and in salad dressings instead of polyunsaturated oils. Monounsaturated fats, like canola and olive oils, help to lower the levels of the LDL cholesterol in your body while polyunsaturated fats lower both HDL and LDL cholesterol.

'I may be a lot heavier than I was when I was thirty, but I would say I'm emotionally much better than I was then, and I live a much healthier life.'

STEPHANIE ALEXANDER

Fat is the most concentrated source of calories in the diet, so when you decrease fat intake you also decrease your calorie intake. To reduce fat in your diet use low-fat dairy products, eat less red meat, eat more fish, choose chicken and vegetarian proteins, trim skin and visible fat from meats and avoid high-fat snack foods and takeaways. Remember, a gram of fat has twice the calories of either carbohydrates or proteins.

Eating more fresh fruit, vegetables and foods containing fibre is essential to a healthy diet. Generous quantities of fruit and vegetables in your diet reduce the risk of heart disease and breast cancer. Foods such as apricots, tomatoes, melons, broccoli and pumpkin are high in vitamins and provide the best protection against these killer diseases.

Eating more foods rich in fibre, particularly the insoluble kind, helps reduce symptoms of chronic constipation. Insoluble fibre absorbs water from the gut making stools bulkier and softer and the elimination of waste easier and faster.

Insoluble fibre has also been linked to a reduction in colon cancer, a disease that kills over 56 000 Americans a year. Two recent studies published in the *New England Journal of Medicine*, however, found that high levels of fruit, vegetables and fibre in the diet failed to prevent the recurrence of potentially cancerous polyps.

Both studies tracked people who had colorectal polyps surgically removed before starting a high-fibre diet. In one study, (Schatzkin *et al.*, 2000) more than 1,900 people over thirty-five were randomly divided into two groups. One group ate a diet of fruit and vegetables and a reduced red meat and fat intake. The other group followed their regular diet. The study showed that after four years the two groups suffered recurring polyps at equal rates of 40 per cent.

The other study (Alberts *et al.*, 2000) included more than 1,300 people aged between forty and eighty. One group of 719 people followed a high-fibre diet while 584 people had a low-fibre regime. As in the previous study, there was no significant difference in the recurrence of polyps in either group. The researchers concluded that although high-fibre diets offer some health advantages they do not prevent the recurrence of colorectal adenomas for up to four years after initial surgery.

The results of these studies were not definitive about the effect of diet on the long-term development of colon cancer.

Fresh fish should be an important part of our diets at menopause. Try to eat two or three servings of fish, such as tuna, herrings, sardines, salmon and trout, each week. These fish are rich in Omega 3 essential fatty acids, substances known to reduce blood clotting, lower blood pressure and protect the body against diabetes, breast cancer and arthritis.

You also need to eat more foods that are rich in phytoestrogen. A high intake of phytoestrogen helps reduce acute menopausal symptoms such as hot flushes, sweats, vaginal dryness and may also reduce the incidence of breast cancer. Phytoestrogen-rich foods include alfalfa, red-clover tea, ginseng tea, soy products, flaxseeds and oil, lentils, beans, carrots, corn, apples, oats, miso soup, celery, fennel, liquorice, rhubarb, dong quai, black cohosh, soy beans and wild yam.

Try to reduce the amount of sugar, salt, caffeine, alcohol, phosphates and saturated fats in your diet. All of these substances have an adverse effect on the levels of calcium in the body, either inhibiting calcium absorption or increasing urinary excretion of calcium.

Sugar is a carbohydrate that provides energy, but no vitamins or proteins. It can contribute to weight gain, blood-sugar swings and increased nutrient excretion.

'Of course, I had menopausal symptoms before then, but, to tell you the truth, there were so many things going on in my life at the time that it's difficult to untangle it all. It was a very torrid period through those years.'

SUE WALKER

Sodium chloride or table salt is an essential nutrient that maintains blood volume and regulates fluid balance. Most of us consume excessive amounts of salt in our daily diets, which causes fluid retention and an increase in calcium excretion. The phosphates in red meat, processed foods and soft drinks also increase calcium excretion.

Caffeine is the stimulant found in coffee, tea, chocolate and soft drinks. It is known to increase excretion of water-soluble vitamins and calcium and causes irritability.

Saturated fats, such as butter, and foods high in fat can raise blood cholesterol levels and increase the risk of heart disease and breast cancer.

Water is essential for good health and a key part of any well-balanced diet. Water facilitates all chemical reactions in your body, helps dissolve solvents, and assists other nutrients to release energy. Try to drink at least six glasses of water each day.

A daily glass of red wine has shown to be beneficial in reducing the risk of heart disease. Red wine is rich in powerful antioxidants called phenols.

There is some debate over the relative benefits of high-carbohydrate and high-protein diets. Australian dietitians tend to promote the healthy diet pyramid, which encourages a diet of reduced fat, moderate protein from low-fat sources and more carbohydrates from breads, pasta, rice, and fruit and vegetable sources.

Supporters of high-protein diets have advocated the benefits of eating high-protein foods, such as fish, meat, poultry, eggs and dairy products, drinking more water and lowering the amount of carbohydrates consumed. This is the diet often recommended by fitness instructors who focus on a weight-training program to build muscles. Muscles need high levels of protein for repairing and strengthening. This type of diet also encourages eating more unrefined, essential oils and fresh fruit, and eating fewer processed oils.

Both high-carbohydrate and high-protein diets have a similar approach to the consumption of processed fats. But these diets differ in the levels of proteins and carbohydrates they recommend.

Some foods, such as potatoes, white bread and white rice quickly increase the body's blood-sugar levels. These foods are described as having a high glycemic index. When your blood sugar increases quickly, the body responds by increasing its insulin levels. High levels of insulin lead to the conversion of excess calories for storage as fat. Low-glycemic foods tend to raise blood sugar levels slowly and maintain this level for longer periods, reducing the urge for food. Examples of low-glycemic foods are: porridge, brans, grain bread and peas.

The *G I Factor* (Miller, 2000) has extensive information on foods for healthy eating and is particularly helpful in suggesting foods for people with diabetes.

Try to eat a variety of low-glycemic carbohydrates, low-fat proteins and very small amounts of fat to assist healthy, sustainable weight loss. Always combine a dietary weight-loss program with exercise to maintain lean muscles and body tone. Your exercise program should include cardiovascular exercise, such as an hour of brisk walking several times a week, and a muscle-toning and strengthening program at least two or three times a week.

The calorie content of foods is important. High-calorie foods have high levels of saturated fat and sugar. Carbohydrates are stored as glycogen and can provide a source of energy for those who participate in endurance exercise. But the body can only store a small level of energy as glycogen – about 1,100 calories worth – compared with the total amount of calories it stores in other forms.

Excess carbohydrates in the body are converted to fat, a process that is encouraged by high-insulin levels. With a low-carbohydrate diet, the body breaks down its glycogen stores for energy first and then breaks down the proteins in muscles to make glucose.

An adequate protein intake is also important, particularly for the elderly and for children. Protein-calorie malnutrition and a prolonged vitamin D deficiency during childhood can have a significant effect on the development of bones and the amount of bone mass obtained in later life. Elderly people with hip fractures are often less nourished than their peers and a high intake of animal proteins may increase the excretion of calcium in the urine.

Ketones are a by-product of muscle-protein breakdown, and there is an increase in the amount of body water lost when the kidney excretes high levels of ketones. Drinking lots of water is essential in a high-protein diet. If the intake of water is low, the body uses its own store of water for ketone excretion in the urine. This leads to temporary weight loss and dehydration.

For sensible weight loss, you need to eat enough carbohydrates to avoid ketone excretion, or ketosis. Eat more low-glycemic carbohydrates that keep your blood sugar at normal levels. These foods include carrots, peas, sweet potatoes, apples, grapefruit, pasta and wholegrain breads.

Dieting with a reduced calorie intake can, in the long-term, lead to an inadequate intake of essential foods such as proteins, vitamins and minerals. Weight loss, as measured on bathroom scales, is often through water loss rather than fat loss.

Increasing the amount of lean muscle and reducing the fat in your body will help to maintain higher metabolic rates. Eat six small meals per day, with each meal combining one carbohydrate and one low-fat protein source. Each meal should provide about 200 calories to give a total daily intake of 1,200 calories.

Stick to appropriate foods that you enjoy and, similarly, an exercise program that is stimulating and can be incorporated into your way of life. We all use the excuse of 'not enough time' to avoid exercise. More often it is a lack of planning and motivation that stops us from exercising. A personal trainer provides both important motivation and a supervised exercise program that gradually increases your levels of strength and fitness.

Drinking small amounts of alcohol can reduce your risk of heart disease, however, epidemiological studies have found that more than two drinks a day slightly increases breast-cancer risk. Women at menopause often find that alcohol, which dilates blood vessels, exacerbates hot flushes.

Rocaltrol, an active form of vitamin D that requires a special prescription, can increase blood calcium levels so women taking this medication need to ensure that their levels of calcium are monitored through a blood test every three months. Some sunblocks can affect the level of vitamin D production in the skin, however, half an hour of sunlight exposure each day maintains the skin's natural vitamin D levels.

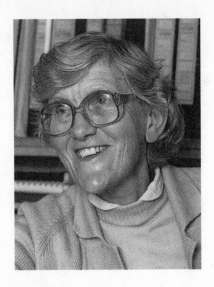

Nancy Millis, AC, MBE, Mag.Sc, Ph.D, Hon.DSc., FTSE, is an emeritus professor and has had an active career since her first academic appointment as a lecturer at the University of Melbourne in 1953. She has been visiting lecturer at the University of Tokyo, and Visiting Research Fellow at Queen Elizabeth College London and the University of Kent. Nancy was awarded a Personal Chair in Microbiology at the University of Melbourne in 1982 and in 1987 was awarded the status of Emeritus Professor. At present she is Chancellor, La Trobe University, consultant to Parks Victoria, Chairman of the Research Advisory Committee, Murray Darling Freshwater Research Centre, and Chairman of the Genetic Manipulations Advisory Committee. She is a member of several other panels involved with scientific research. In 1977 she was awarded an MBE and became a Fellow of the Australian Academy of Technological Sciences. In 1987 she became an Honorary Life Member of the Australian Society for Microbiology and in 1990 she became a Companion in the Order of Australia (AC). The Victorian Government awarded her a Victorian Achiever Award in 1992.

Nancy Millis

As far as I was concerned, menopause was a biological event. It was a bloody nuisance while it lasted, and when it was over I thought, Thank goodness for that. And that was it; I just got on with it.

As a biologist, you are perhaps a little better informed than the average person, so you say to yourself, This is one of the things that goes with being female as distinct from being male. Our periods might be necessary, but they certainly are a nuisance and, as far as I'm concerned, stopping them for good is a damn good idea.

As far as dealing with menopause, I guess there isn't a lot to tell. I'm the sort of person who's always got on with the job at hand. It was the same with menopause. It was simply an event that passed by and while it did I just got on with doing what I was doing previously.

There is no virtue in being a woman. For many of us periods have always been a chore, leaving us feeling dreadful for the first day or so every month. I was never at my very best around that time of the month, but it didn't worry me unduly. I don't think I was really any different from the next person. It just happens to be the way you're made, and I was lucky.

As for growing older, well, one is always growing older – as it is quite clear I am now – so I don't take a great deal of notice of that. But there are things I notice about myself that I can no longer do. For example, I don't hear as well as I used to do. In large gatherings, like functions or meetings, I've noticed that women's voices are very hard to hear. I had a scan for my hearing range. I hear quite well up to a particular wavelength and then, boom, my hearing collapses. So there are certain sounds I simply do not hear, which is a nuisance.

Similarly, my eyesight is not as good as it used to be, and I can't read some things, such as slides in a presentation. That's also irritating to live with. But I can still read. I just need to have very good light now.

I can't really pinpoint any stage where I experienced any great changes between pre- and postmenopause. I've noticed that I've put on a bit of weight around the middle in the last four or five years, but before that I was pretty much the same shape as I had always been.

I used to play sport when I was younger, but I stopped all that around my late thirties. I don't think I lack any energy. I still garden and walk a lot, but I don't carry heavy loads up hill as well as I used to.

I don't think the changes I've experienced are particularly related to menopause; it's just age. You live with all sorts of changes. I don't believe there's any particular feature of menopause that has changed my outlook.

I think as we get older and our lives change that it's important to have interests to pursue. I continued to be a salaried university teacher until I retired at sixty-five. Lots of people say that if you are still active you should continue beyond the retirement age. Personally, I don't agree with that. I believe that by the time you reach retirement it's high time you got out so that somebody younger can take your place.

I was reasonably on top of what I was doing and could have easily continued teaching beyond sixty-five. But when I stopped teaching I still had a number of tasks to do, mostly in the area of genetics. I also had a great interest in water and water-related issues. I've been on a number of councils, committees and boards of management and, in those roles, I've continued my interest in science. But it's not been as a hands-on player.

The philosophy I adopt is that people will soon enough stop asking you to do things if you louse them up. They won't ask you a second time. So if people ask me to something and they're satisfied with the result, they may ask me again. If they do, that's great, and if they don't, well, that's okay too.

As far as having a regular health check goes, I must confess that I'm not as vigilant as I should be. I recognise the value of regular checks, but I find I haven't got time to have them, which is wicked. I should make time, but I don't. The only things I have checked regularly are my eyes. I have to look after them a bit otherwise I won't have them.

After my episode with cancer when I was forty, the doctors recommended that I should keep having regular checks. I kept that up for around seven years, but that all happened so long ago now.

When I did have cancer – it was quite a radical treatment in those days – after six weeks of radiation treatment I told the doctor that I'd planned to take a holiday. I remember him saying what a good idea that was . . . until I told him that the destination was Tanzania. Then he didn't think it was such a wise move.

But I went off to Tanzania anyway and had a wonderful six-week holiday. When I came back I was in remission.

When I was in my fifties – which was a long time ago now – there was very little talk of hormone replacement therapy. It almost didn't exist.

I went to school with one of the pioneers in this field, Jean Hailes, and I had great admiration for the job she did. But it was a real uphill job at the time she began her work. Nobody was interested. Hot flushes were thought to be nothing more than a bar-room joke. It was a struggle to establish that menopause was a real problem for a lot of women.

Although I was lucky enough to avoid any difficulties during my menopause, I realise that it was simply a part of my biological luck. But for other women it is very difficult, and I would advise anyone who was struggling with symptoms to seek the help of the experts.

I'm not a medical expert in this field, I'm simply a biological scientist, but I have very real reservations about many of the so-called natural approaches to medical science. That's not to say they have no basis or that they should be dismissed totally. But I have a good deal of reservation about any approach when the data are really not well prepared or well presented.

Given this, I think if I were suffering from any adverse symptoms of menopause I would choose hormone replacement therapy as my first option. I'm pretty sceptical of the herbal purists. Of course, herbs do have a place, but I personally would not make them my first choice.

I'm reserving my final view on hormone replacement therapy because I don't think anyone at this time has provided what I would consider to be enough statistical evidence to support or refute its worth. I like to keep an open mind on the matter, but I do not believe it is a potent cause of cancer.

There are people who are quite wary of hormone replacement therapy. I can only advise women who want to know more to make sure they go to a clinic that specialises in this field. That way you have every expectation that you will receive the very best and latest advice.

Chapter Thirteen
Common problems and questions

Hot flushes and night sweats. Vaginal dryness. Bladder infections and incontinence. Heavy periods and bleeding. Palpitations and anxiety. Migraines. Weight gain. Sexuality. Stress.

Hot flushes and night sweats

Many women wonder why they have hot flushes and sweats when their friends do not, and vice versa. As with morning sickness and pregnancy, if you have not experienced it then you may tend to think it is 'all in the mind' of those who do experience it. If you have had significant nausea with pregnancy, you will know that you are not imagining it – it is very real. As with morning sickness, hot flushes may be only mild, and you may be able cope with them without any need for medication. Alternatively, they may be severe. Only you can be the judge of how much they affect your well-being.

Hot flushes and night sweats are the most characteristic symptoms of menopause. They are caused by the lower levels of oestrogen associated with ovarian failure, and possibly also the change from high to lower levels of oestrogen. The effects of oestrogen deficiency are mediated through a complex system within the brain that is primed by the presence of oestrogen. The flushes are the result of withdrawal of oestrogen from specific areas within the brain.

There is no difference in the oestrogen levels of those who have hot flushes and those women who do not experience them. There may be a critical level of oestrogen for each woman that will determine whether she has, or continues to have, hot flushes, or whether she does not. Eventually, it seems that the body adjusts to the lower oestrogen levels.

Most women do stop having hot flushes and night sweats. How long this will take is impossible to predict with any certainty, but in most women these symptoms disappear in a few months.

'When I was in my twenties, I thought by the time I was fifty I would probably be retired. I am now sixty-one and far from being retired. With my health intact, I believe I will still be going strong at eighty.'

DIANA ABRUZZI

Oestrogen effectively reduces hot flushes and night sweats in most women. Hot flushes and night sweats can significantly affect the quality of life and feeling of well-being of some women. Whether a woman decides to take oestrogen replacement therapy to reduce hot flushes is an individual decision. Hot flushes, though unpleasant, are not life threatening. There may be women who have other concurrent, or previous, medical illnesses where oestrogen replacement therapy is contraindicated. It is important to discuss the advantages and disadvantages of taking hormone replacement therapy with your doctor. Ultimately, it should be your decision.

Some of the women in our interviews, for example, Stephanie Alexander and Barbara Champion, were advised to try hormone replacement therapy and found it beneficial; others wanted to try alternative therapies. Some were not at all happy about being told to take it, and some had side effects, or found that it made little difference to their overall health.

There are no hard and fast rules. You need to make your own decision after you have discussed the issue thoroughly with your doctor.

There is no reason why you cannot try it for two to three months if you are uncertain about whether it will help you. There is also no length of time for which it should be taken. You can stop it at any time, particularly if you are only using it to alleviate symptoms. If you are taking it for other reasons, for example, osteoporosis, then there may be an alternative therapy that is equally beneficial for your condition. Hormone replacement therapy, however, is the cheapest medication for the prevention and treatment of osteoporosis, particularly in women who have not had a fracture.

Many women, for various reasons, do not want to use hormone replacement therapy for menopausal symptoms. Progestins, which are synthetically made progesterone-like medications, can reduce hot flushes in some women. Some of the women we interviewed preferred to use various phytoestrogen products, for example, Ita Buttrose. These can be useful for mild hot flushes.

Other women have tried Chinese herbs, creams containing progesterone, or derivatives from wild yams to treat their menopausal symptoms. Although anecdotally these treatments appear to work, not enough research has been done to evaluate their true effects, or whether they are safe to use over a long period. It is important to consider whether you are using a product that actually contains what it is reported to contain, whether the expense justifies its use, and whether you have considered any possible short- and long-term side effects. No product, whether manufactured or 'natural', is free from possible side effects.

Vaginal dryness

Vaginal dryness is another characteristic symptom of menopause, but it may not become a problem until several years after menopause begins. Vaginal dryness arises as a result of oestrogen deficiency. There is a gradual thinning of the vaginal tissue due to a decrease in the blood flow and general lack of oestrogen action on the tissues. On examination, your doctor will see red, inflamed, sensitive tissue, which is quite different from the pink moist tissue when the vagina is well supplied with oestrogen. Intercourse becomes painful and the vagina becomes susceptible to infections such as thrush. Sometimes the vulva also becomes itchy and has a burning feeing.

Local treatment in the form of an oestrogen-containing pessary, tablet, cream or vaginal ring will successfully treat the problem. Usually, there needs to be an intensive treatment every night for two weeks, then the effects are maintained by twice-weekly use. It is important to treat any likely infections before starting to use oestrogen creams or pessaries. Occasionally, an infection may develop after treatment starts because the acidity in the vagina changes and promotes the growth of bacteria. This will need to be treated.

'I have worked in life not necessarily to change the world but to change the little bit of the world, where I and other feminists can make a difference. That's my passion, and it's my passion that keeps me going.'

JOAN KIRNER

These local oestrogen treatments generally do not have any effects on the rest of the body. As a precaution, women who use vaginal oestrogens continuously for long periods may be given a 'progestin challenge'. This involves a short course of twelve days of oral progestins to see if there is bleeding from the uterus after stopping the tablets. This is called a withdrawal bleed. It means that the vaginal oestrogen has had an effect on the lining of the uterus or endometrium. Progestins may need to be given more regularly if withdrawal bleeding does occur. Vulval irritation, such as itchiness at night, can be caused by conditions such as eczema or drying and general thinning of the skin from ageing. Simple regimes, such as avoiding soaps and other irritants, may be all that is needed. If the condition is persistent, a mild cortisone cream with or without a fungal cream used intermittently can be helpful.

These symptoms may also be caused by lichen sclerosis, which is an autoimmune condition that particularly affects the vulval area but is also seen occasionally in other areas of the body. A small biopsy is usually needed to confirm the diagnosis and to plan long-term treatment.

This condition causes a whitening of the vulval skin, as well as gradual thinning and eventual loss of the contour of the vulval tissue. It usually needs treatment with cortisone creams to control the symptoms. Lichen sclerosis may or may not produce any symptoms. Your doctor will diagnose the condition during a check-up.

Women who have an active and regular sex life have fewer vaginal problems. 'Use it or lose it' is an oft-quoted saying that also applies in this context.

Women should understand that at this time of their lives their male partners may have sexual difficulties. Impotence in men gradually increases with age and erectile dysfunction is common.

Bladder infections and incontinence

Women may also have symptoms that are related to the bladder, such as frequency in passing urine, recurrent bladder infections (cystitis) or incontinence. These symptoms may, in part, be related to oestrogen deficiency and, in part, to ageing. The prevalence of urinary incontinence in women in their menopause has been variously quoted as between 8 and 52 per cent.

The two main types of incontinence are stress incontinence, when women cough or sneeze and 'wet themselves', and urge incontinence, when they feel the urge to pass urine and find they are unable to hold on. Some women experience features of both.

Urge incontinence occurs because the main bladder muscle, the detrusor muscle, is overactive or hypersensitive even to a small amount of urine. Retraining the bladder to hold more urine can help, as well as trying some local oestrogen therapy. More research needs to be done in this area to determine the effectiveness of oestrogen therapy. Other drug therapy can also be very useful for this problem, as it helps the bladder relax and reduces the urgent feeling.

Stress incontinence is the result of an imbalance between the pressure in the bladder and the pressure in the urethra. Weakness of the supporting pelvic floor muscles aggravates the problem. Exercises to strengthen the pelvic floor muscles can be beneficial and, if done regularly and effectively, for 60 per cent of women can largely resolve the problem.

Heavy periods and bleeding

About 50 per cent of women will notice that their periods become heavier in their early to mid forties. This problem may be superimposed on a lifetime tendency to have heavy menstrual bleeding, or it may be a new problem. There is much research being conducted about the cause of perimenopausal bleeding. Often heavy bleeding is caused by a hormonal imbalance. However, in some women the problem may be due to abnormal enzyme function within the glands and blood vessels of the endometrium.

As menopause approaches, there are some cycles in which ovulation does not occur. This results in too much oestrogen and not enough progesterone to balance it. The lining thickens and breaks down excessively causing prolonged, heavy bleeding. Medications containing progestins, for example, Provera or Primolut N, are given to women to help control the bleeding. They may be given when the bleeding occurs or as a preventive treatment during the menstrual cycle to lighten the menstrual loss. Other drugs that may be used include medications that help stop bleeding and include the antiprostaglandins, such as Naprosyn, or a newer treatment called Cyklokapron, which is given for four days after the period starts.

A very good alternative medication that can be effective in regulating the cycle and controlling bleeding is the oral contraceptive pill. It will often be also useful for treating hot flushes in women who are still having periods, but are experiencing symptoms. The pill is generally more effective in achieving regular, lighter bleeding and controlling hot flushes than hormone replacement therapy during the perimenopausal phase. The pill can be used for women up to their early fifties as long as there are no risk factors for thrombosis and they are not smoking. It is also effective in controlling some benign breast diseases, such as breast cysts.

The standard oral contraceptive pill can be used, but there are now low-dose oral contraceptive pills that are suitable for perimenopausal women. These pills contain only 20 micrograms of ethinyloestradiol, a level of oestrogen that was used previously for hormone replacement therapy. Microgynon 20 and Loette are the most common low-dose pills available.

Some women who continue to have heavy bleeding despite medical treatment will need surgical intervention. This may involve a 'curette' where the lining is thinned down by scraping the tissue away, and may be just a temporary solution.

Other women may be advised to have an endometrial ablation, where the lining is scraped away more extensively so that the underlying glands that build up the lining during each cycle are removed. This may be successful, in varying degrees, in 70 to 80 per cent of women.

As a last resort, a hysterectomy, the removal of the uterus, will be the ultimate method of stopping bleeding. Many women are quite happy to have this procedure and have no regrets. Others feel it reduces their perception of themselves as feminine. The decision should therefore not be taken lightly. It is a major operation and does have possible complications. Discuss the issue fully with your doctor and seek a second opinion if you wish.

Palpitations and anxiety

Palpitations and anxiety can occur together or separately. Some women experience disturbing palpitations before they ever have a hot flush. A number of women will undergo extensive tests on their heart before it is realised that the cause is menopause. Some women are woken suddenly at night feeling panicked and anxious. They may have had an episode of sweating while they were sleeping and the resulting disturbance of the cardiovascular system causes a racing heart. Usually an explanation by your doctor and their reassurance that there is nothing serious happening with the heart is helpful to most women who have this symptom. Hormone replacement therapy may also help.

Migraines

Migraines can plague some women all their lives, but they commonly start around puberty. Migraines are usually caused by a multitude of factors: genes, the environment, foods, chemicals, and hormonal changes. Some women find that they occur at particular phases of their cycles, such as premenstrually. Changes in hormonal levels are implicated in this situation. Hormone levels may be within the normal range, but the change from higher to lower levels or visa versa may be the precipitating factor. Oestrogen and progesterone are the hormones most often implicated, but prostaglandins produced by the uterus before menstruation are also considered to play a role.

Sometimes hormone therapy helps in migraines that increase after menopause. When a woman suffers from menopausal migraines, transdermal patches are often used because they tend to maintain blood levels more consistently than oral medications. Other more specific migraine treatments should also be tried, as well as preventive treatments if migraines are occurring weekly or more often.

Weight gain

Along with hot flushes, weight gain is probably the main complaint of women at menopause. Some women are convinced that hormone replacement therapy is the cause, but this is uncommonly the case. We have some very good evidence from well-designed clinical trials, such as the PEPI study in the US, that hormone replacement therapy is not an important contributing factor to weight gain at menopause.

The PEPI study was conducted over three years and compared women using hormone replacement with women using a placebo medication in a randomised, double-blind study. None of the subjects knew which substance they were using for the duration of the trial. The researchers evaluated a few different effects of hormone replacement therapy, for example, on bones, cholesterol and weight gain. In both groups of women, those on active and those on inactive treatment, there was weight gain, but the hormone replacement therapy inactive group actually gained 1 to 2 kilograms less than the placebo or inactive group.

A number of factors probably contribute to weight gain at menopause. These include a declining metabolic rate with ageing, a more sedentary way of life, intake of more calories overall than are needed, and less lean muscle tissue as opposed to fatty tissue. Very occasionally, an underactive thyroid gland, more common at this stage of life, may be a factor. Body contour and shape changes do occur, with an increase in abdominal fat. This appears to be a physiological change, but may be contributed to by an overall increase in body weight.

Many of the women we interviewed said that weight gain was a problem – and all of those interviewed are very active women. These women have adopted very sensible strategies. They realise they need to eat sensibly and adjust their food intake to lower levels with more fruits and vegetables and less fatty, high calorie foods. Several have introduced exercise programs, or extended them.

The principal aim for women who are concerned about weight gain should be to seek a healthy eating pattern (planning this may need some help from a good dietician) and a regular exercise regime with a combination of aerobic fitness and muscle strengthening and toning. A quick weight loss diet is not recommended. Remember that being in the healthy weight range (and being happy) is more important than having a stick-like figure. It may be impossible to get back to size ten again, but size twelve or fourteen is very acceptable if this gives you a body mass index of twenty-five or lower. Allow yourself some treats of the foods you really like, but eat these in smaller quantities, or learn to eat less the next day to compensate for today's overindulgence.

Never say, 'Tomorrow is when I'll start.' Tomorrow you will probably think the same as you do today. Start straight away, but don't be hard on yourself if you give in to temptations such as either not exercising when you should or indulging in foods that you know you should not have had. Just keep a positive outlook and maintain an easy-to-follow program that focuses on what you like doing, particularly with exercise. If you are unable to fit it all into one week because you have other commitments, aim to resume your exercise the following week or as soon as you can.

Sexuality

As discussed in the chapter on sexuality, sexual responses, enjoyment and desire may change around menopause. Men and women in long-term relationships show a decline in the frequency of sex. Being physically unwell at menopause and 'out of sorts' and moody is often the result of the lack of sleeping due to hot sweats and flushes. Fatigue and difficulty in coping with everyday life takes its toll. There may not be enough emotional or physical energy left at the end of the day for an active sex life. Treating yourself and your partner to regular weekends or holidays away in a relaxing environment may be important for both of you to rejuvenate an intimate relationship.

'I think it is another sneaky trick of nature that it is not until you get to fifty or so that you can afford to think, Well, I spent all those years doing things for other people, what am I going to do for me?'

TONIA TODMAN

One of the problems for women in their sixties and seventies is finding a suitable partner. It is not that they are not interested, but that they lack suitable and available men. In addition, certain medications may affect libido. The SSRIs, the group of drugs that are commonly used for depression at any age, interfere with both desire and orgasm. It is important to discuss any of these problems with your doctor.

Stress

Most women in their forties and fifties have very busy lives. They may be juggling careers, have adolescent children or elderly parents to support and care for. Many events are taking place in their lives at a time when physical and psychological changes are occurring. During the perimenopausal phase, which can last for four or five years, or longer, there can be a state of relative 'hormone chaos' with the fluctuation of oestrogen, progesterone and testosterone levels. Stressful daily events can aggravate the symptoms that women experience or make it more difficult to cope. Huge life stresses, such as coping with death, severe illness or separation and divorce can precipitate some women into menopause.

Many women complain of excessive fatigue and tiredness. While this can be the consequence of poor sleep in response to some menopausal symptoms such as hot flushes, stress can cause very significant fatigue and lack of energy.

Several of the women we interviewed were under stress. Sources of their stress included demanding jobs, death of a spouse, separation or divorce, coping with children without a supporting partner, and cancer. These situations reflect the lives of many women at this time of life. It is interesting and informative to see how different women tackled their situations. Sue Carr coped with her mother's death from cancer. Ita Buttrose had a very demanding business in difficult economic times.

Generally, they aimed to improve their lives by paying more attention to their diet, trying to extend their exercise program, or using vitamins and alternative medicines. They often visualised themselves as being in control. They sought help, but only used the advice if it suited their personal outlook on life.

One valuable strategy that many of those interviewed used was to override negative feelings as much as they could. Although some were struggling with physical and emotional symptoms as well as many challenges and difficulties with their work, they tried to maintain a positive attitude. They endeavoured to live life in the present, and kept on making plans for the future.

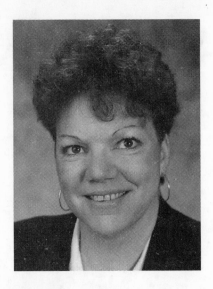

Barbara Champion is Chief Executive Officer of the Playground and Recreation Association of Victoria. She has an executive history in local government as a councillor for the City of Melbourne 1991–93 and as Chief Commissioner for the City of Maribyrnong during the amalgamation process. Prior to 1994 Barbara worked in the employment sector as the manager of the Central Community Employment Association, after many years as a teacher and Policy and Program Director in the Ministry of Education. Her experience ranges across years of active leadership and involvement in a number of community-based education, arts and health organisations in inner city areas. She was recently appointed the Deputy Chancellor of Victoria University.

Barbara Champion

My general pattern of life hasn't changed, I suppose, in thirty years. As long as I can remember, I have always been busier than most, and that, no doubt, has been to accommodate my need to engage with people and be involved with social causes of interest to me.

What I find generally is that as I get older I don't seem to have the same amount of energy I had as a younger woman, but I'm not sure that this is due to menopause. The ageing process, as well as carrying extra weight and not being as physically active as I should, may be the cause of lower energy levels compared with thirty years ago. I enjoy eight hours sleep a night these days whereas in my earlier years as a teacher I would exist on four hours for weeks on end, or so it seemed!

The changes that did come about as a result of menopause surprised me to an extent, in that I view myself as a well-informed person, but I found I was surprisingly ignorant of a number of health-related issues. I had never spent any time thinking about menopause, I suppose because there seemed to be more interesting things to think about. Perhaps too my cultural and family upbringing has contributed to my practice of not taking time to ponder the implications of ageing. I think that people of my parents' generation, with few exceptions, who lived through war and depression, did not focus on their personal health because in those years their priorities were to get on with living, no matter how poorly they might have felt. I was brought up in this environment and my oldest friends, with whom I trained to be a teacher, would have a similar perspective. As a matter of course we don't reflect on our health beyond what requires urgent attention. I do notice that younger women seem to spend considerably more time on their personal health than those of my generation. Young women seem to think about what they eat, what they do, all aspects of their lifestyle, whereas my generation was a bit inclined just to get on with it. I do think the knowledge we have today of the importance of exercise and diet is much greater than it was when I was younger, but even so I think that younger women have different attitudes from those of my generation.

My mother was a feminist who had four children, but I cannot recall any conversation with her *ever* about menopause, which people who knew my mother would find most interesting, given that she was a great conversationalist, an extremely competent and well-informed woman with significant skills in both her professional and personal life. We just didn't talk about those kinds of subjects. She worked for many of her adult years, and there is no doubt that these were the happiest and most fulfilling years of her life. I enjoyed her as a mother enormously. In fact, that she didn't initiate discussion on what seemed to be very personal issues seemed to me as a younger person to be one of her strengths. Predictably, I would very much like to discuss some of these issues with her now.

I don't have any children and in a sense the whole reproductive issue has never been of any significant interest for me, probably because I wasn't personally engaged in it.

I can remember conducting my first graduation ceremony at the university in 2000. It was a particularly difficult day for me as I seemed to be overcome with hot flushes every moment. Whether it was a sense of anxiousness, or the fact that I had to stand up for two hours and make every student feel like they were the most important student in the ceremony, while losing a lot of blood, I'm not sure, but I remember thinking, I wonder if our Chancellor has ever felt anything like this during graduations. You go on, don't you? I mean, I wasn't going to faint. I had a desk behind me just in case I did, but you also don't talk about it to your colleagues, especially given that most of them at this level are male.

I don't seem to have many symptoms in menopause compared with some others, even though I do now take a mild form of hormone replacement therapy. Some years ago I was fortunate to find a wonderful general practitioner, and I trust her judgement enormously. She considers all the information available prior to reaching any conclusion about the appropriate course of action. She and I came to the view that it was worthwhile taking hormones for a few years, and that has been terrific. Certainly I have felt more invigorated.

I also use soy products as much as I can to supplement the hormones in a natural way. I'm a regular drinker of soy milk. My diet has changed over the years, not due to menopause necessarily but from the growing knowledge of the dangers of fat in the diet.

I think that managing your health in the optimum way requires a lot of time and energy, which I don't have. I've got work to do, meetings to run, and holidays to organise!

I have a number of female friends about my own age – between fifty and fifty-five – and that's a pretty common age for menopause, and we discuss menopause occasionally. I am fortunate to have an extremely supportive partner.

Obviously I did feel that I was suffering at the time of the decision to take additional hormones, as I went back repeatedly to the doctor, saying that I didn't feel well. Whether it's affected my work and output, it's hard to say. For a long time I've been very much in control of my time in relation to my work and I have had more flexibility than many other women.

Not having the responsibilities of children has meant that I can live my life as I choose. Not that menopausal women have generally got young children, but a number do, and how they manage sometimes in terms of energy levels I have absolutely no idea.

I was the Chief Commissioner of the City of Maribyrnong during the beginning of my menopause – from 1995 to 1998 – and I don't think that my work was affected, possibly because I was the boss and able to have considerable control over my working time.

I get concerned occasionally about growing old, but as I don't feel any older than previously, except on the occasions when I get very tired, it's not something that I think much about. This may have something to do with not having had children. It may also be due to living with a man who is nine years older than me. However I am aware that my hair is not as thick as it used to be, and that drives me mad – I loved my thick straight hair. When I can't do something because of my age I guess I will focus on ageing more than I do now.

I do notice that I can have significant mood changes. I would not have described myself as a moody person, but I find sometimes that the tiniest matter can annoy and upset me significantly. I've also gained a little weight. Whether it's to do with menopause or because I eat too much and don't exercise enough, I'm not sure.

Menopause has possibly reduced my sexual drive, but I think it's very changeable. I don't know how long it has been different, and I don't know how long it will last. I'm nearly fifty-three, and I guess I've been in my menopause for about four or five years. I imagine that my doctor will say in another year or so, 'Well, I think we ought to reconsider your hormone replacement therapy,' because she doesn't think I should be on it for too long.

Life hasn't changed in any significant way due to menopause. I enjoy what I do, I love my family and friends, and don't imagine any aspect of my life, beyond winning Tattslotto (to which I don't subscribe), could be much better. I have a very comfortable life, and I'm very fortunate. There doesn't seem to me to have been any big turning point.

I have regular mammograms and pap smears and believe we are very fortunate to be able to have those health screenings.

I think there are some differences in my life from ten years ago, but I don't think that this is due to menopause, but simply growing older and hopefully gaining some wisdom along the way.

My mother used to say that all girls, in fact, all people should learn biology. I never learned biology at school, so when I'm considering my own ignorance about how the body works I understand why she would have thought this. Perhaps the next generation will be better informed from an earlier age about the changes caused by menopause.

Chapter Fourteen
Sexuality

Changes in sexuality as we age. Reasons for decreased sexual drive.
Effects of changing oestrogen levels on the body. The role of testosterone.
Some ideas for improving your sex life.

During the perimenopausal and postmenopausal years, sexual functioning for many women and their partners does not alter significantly. Most women and men continue to be sexually active in their middle years and maintain their interest well into their sixties and seventies.

With older age, the availability of a suitable and interested sexual partner may be an inhibiting factor. For some women, sexuality may be affected by personal physical or psychological illness, their partner's medical problems, or difficulties arising from marital conflict. Some women may feel that the hormonal changes of menopause affect their libido. At the same time, their partners may be experiencing problems with their sexual ability and performance. As a result, there may be widely variable sexual functioning in women and men at this stage of their lives.

Age-related changes occur in women, which are not specifically the result of an alteration in hormonal levels associated with menopause. There may be a decrease in sexual drive and desire, and changes in body image. Some women have negative feelings about developing wrinkles, grey hair and gaining weight. Other women may work hard to maintain a youthful image. Others just accept these changes as inevitable, they are able to comfortably adjust to the changes that age brings. Expectations and beliefs about sexuality in men and women at mid-life may influence their relationship. They may feel that sex is just for vibrant young men and women.

'I'm divorced. I live with my two teenage children and my dog and cat. And I certainly don't walk around having sexual thoughts about them. If there was a bloke around the place I might feel a bit more sexy, but it's a bit hard without one.'

ITA BUTTROSE

Some women lack interest in, or are bored with, their partner. Other women may have had little interest in the sexual aspect of their marriage prior to menopause. The physical changes of menopause and ageing may contribute to a further decline in their libido. They may seek help and advice not for themselves, but 'to please their partner'.

Resolving marital conflict or other stresses may be necessary for a successful sexual relationship. Most marriages have episodes where there are difficulties in the relationship. The person you marry at twenty-five will be in some ways the same, but in other ways different by the time you are fifty. The excitement of being 'in love' early in married life allows many people to accept or ignore faults in their partners.

Once the initial romance fades, we tend to see our partner in a more realistic way, and this may affect the sexual relationship. The satisfaction with and frequency of sexual contact may alter as couples become more familiar with each other. By the time some couples reach middle age, both may be accepting of less frequent sexual intercourse. Problems usually arise in a marriage if one of the partners has a greater sexual drive and desire than the other. Many women seek help at the instigation of their partner, not necessarily for themselves. Other women seek help believing that the sexual dysfunction in their marriage is their problem, when it may be because their partner is having difficulties.

Problems with libido in perimenopausal and postmenopausal women should not be considered simply a matter of hormonal changes – many forces play a role. There is no doubt, however, that the physical changes and hormonal changes as a result of ageing do alter sexual responses in women. But there is great variability from one woman to another.

Menopause is associated with a significant decline in the production of oestrogen from the ovary, although women who are overweight may still produce higher levels of oestrogen than thinner women. The adrenal gland produces a hormone called andro-stenedione, which is converted to a weaker form of oestrogen in fatty tissue. This form of oestrogen may allow some women to maintain a satisfactory level of vaginal lubrication. There *are* some advantages to being overweight.

In general, however, oestrogen deficiency results in gradual thinning of the vaginal lining and a change in the acidity within the vagina. As a result, there may be an increased susceptibility to non-sexually transmitted vaginal infections. Vaginal lubrication, which depends on a strong oestrogen effect, may decrease and intercourse can become painful.

Oestrogen influences many areas of a woman's body, including the breasts and skin. As a woman ages, she may notice an abnormal increase in skin and nipple sensitivity. It may be unpleasant to be touched and certainly not sexually stimulating. Oestrogen, however, may not play a strong role in sexual drive.

As well as changes in oestrogen levels with menopause, there is a gradual decline in the production of testosterone from the ovary in much the same way that there is a gradual decline in testosterone levels in men as they age. What role testosterone plays in sexual drive in women has not been clearly defined. Testosterone replacement therapy use in women who experience a natural menopause is controversial.

Young women who have had an oophorectomy, or surgical removal of their ovaries, benefit from oestrogen and testosterone replacement therapy for maintaining sexual drive and libido. But research using testosterone in women who have had oophorectomies is selective. Whether the findings of these studies can be extrapolated to normal postmenopausal women is controversial.

All aspects of sexuality, marital relationships, and other life stresses should be considered in postmenopausal women who have had a natural menopause before testosterone replacement therapy is used. Some medical drugs, such as antidepressants, may interfere with libido, and women who are using them and have a low libido should take this up with their doctor.

'Now I find that people are beginning to see me as an

"older" woman when it doesn't seem all that long ago

that I thought of myself simply as an attractive woman.'

ELAINE CANTY

Oral, transdermal, or topical oestrogen therapies will help with vaginal dryness and the sensory skin changes. Vaginal lubricants – jellies and oils – are also useful.

Making an effort to create a romantic environment, spending time alone without children, going on regular holidays together, stimulating sexual fantasies, and relieving boredom by altering sexual activities will all help to rekindle a fading sexual desire.

If there is a persistent problem with sexual dysfunction, then seeking advice from a sex therapist may be useful. Many women (and men) are unaware that low sexual desire may stem from an upbringing that has considered sex to be undesirable, except for having children. Fears about pregnancy may have inhibited some women early in their sexual lives, and they may never have learnt to relax and enjoy it.

Many couples are concerned about the frequency of intercourse compared with their view of its frequency between other couples. Once a day may suit some couples, once a week some, and once a month, or rarely, others. If each person in the relationship is happy about the situation then that is normal for them. It is when one person, or both, are dissatisfied that difficulties arise.

> 'I still have a great desire to be feminine and participate in life with energy and enthusiasm. You could say that the "hormones may not be dancing" but other feelings and a sense of security provide me with energy and desire.'
>
> LORETO DAVEY

Improving communication, and sometimes reaching a compromise, as with other aspects of married life, is important. Each person should consider their own needs and then the needs of their partner. In many marriages a satisfactory sexual life provides a good basis for a happy marriage. But in some marriages couples are very happy without a regular sexual relationship. As long as both partners are happy, it must be right for them.

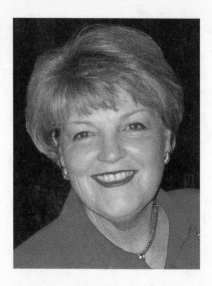

Loreto Davey started her career in nursing at
St. Vincent's Hospital. She expanded her experience
and business knowledge with courses in health
administration, marketing and business planning.
These achievements have allowed her to excel in her
profession. Loreto has been Director of Nursing at
Vimy House Private Hospital, Chief Executive
Officer and Director of Nursing at Cotham Private
Hospital, Cliveden Hill Private Hospital and
Coorana Private Hospital, and is currently Chief
Executive Officer and Director of Nursing at
Swinburne University Hospital, Hawthorn. She
enjoys the challenge of transforming an organisation's vision into reality. Loreto has also played a
significant role in community affairs, having been a
councillor and elected Mayor of Boroondara for two
consecutive terms.

Loreto Davey

Menopause. It was a little difficult to determine the exact time for me as I had a hysterectomy before I was forty. My menopausal symptoms were gradual and almost innocuous in the early days. I do recall being tired, and experiencing hot flushes, and my capacity to cope was challenged. By this I mean that what I would have regarded as a simple task seemed more difficult. My symptoms included palpitations, lack of energy, loss of bladder control and lower libido. As these symptoms persisted I did in fact seek medical advice and was diagnosed as premenopausal. I was given treatment primarily to relieve the symptoms that caused me personal embarrassment. I felt that I needed to be in control of myself if I could, and if this required medical assistance then that was appropriate.

For women, menopause is unavoidable as it is part of our natural physiology. What is important I believe is how we handle this phase of our lives. I sought the best advice available. My consultation with my gynaecologist – who was a specialist in menopause – was comprehensive and she discussed with me and asked me to consider the available options. After due consideration and more reading and research I decided to use a hormone replacement therapy, or more specifically a patch. This treatment did relieve my symptoms and I felt a great deal better, more relaxed and comfortable, however I was also aware that I was gaining weight. This I did not enjoy. Because of the weight gain I only used the patches for a couple of years and then tried some herbal products with quite satisfactory results.

That was twenty-odd years ago. Over the past twenty years I have experienced some of the best and most enjoyable challenges my professional career has offered. I have not had a great deal of time to dwell on how I felt, as I enjoyed the challenges. However, I may have discussed some of the issues with close friends.

What was happening to me during my menopause and the ten years leading up to it wasn't something you sat down and discussed around the table. But it was reassuring to know that other people experienced similar symptoms. I do recall asking my mother how she dealt with menopause and how long it went on for, and I was surprised when she responded that she couldn't even remember it – she had reared seven children – but I can remember it happening to her. I don't know that her generation of women would have talked about it at all. How things have changed, and for the better, as today menopause has a higher profile and is discussed more fully. It is discussed in magazines and journals, at public meetings by eminent medical staff, on the radio, and the internet, and there are a variety of natural therapies available.

During my premenopausal phase, at forty, I was appointed a Director of Nursing. This was my first real challenge in a management role. I was on a very steep and quick learning curve with this new position. It was during this time that I started to notice some symptoms which doctors put down to stress. But I did not feel it was stress, and in hindsight it was probably related to the symptoms of menopause. This does not mean that I have not experienced stress, for I have had to learn to deal with that. Learning to relax and identifying what const-itutes relaxation for me is something I have explored and developed. One of my greatest pleasures is to enjoy the skills and talents of others – this may be in craft, fashion design, art – or relaxing on the beach. I have enjoyed and been energised by the roles I have experienced.

One of the greatest challenges, I believe, is motherhood, with all its responsibilities. It is a busy, demanding and rewarding experience to see and enjoy the development of your children into adulthood. I was fortunate to share this experience with my husband, and have his support. Balancing the needs of a family and a career is perhaps the biggest challenge of all for mothers. I believe this dual role probably diluted to some extent the impact that my menopausal symptoms were having on me physically.

I suppose for me it was the good old Irish coming out in me – this is not going to beat me, I have got to work through this. That is probably what drove me.

In the years from forty to fifty-five, the changes I went through didn't seem to have an effect on the work I was doing. If I look back, I think there were times when I put too much effort into work. I should have made more time for holidays. However, I felt I had to keep on going. Professionally my role as a hospital executive and 'trouble shooter' was demanding and limited opportunities for leisure.

It was during these years that I experienced migraines, once again aligned to stress. My mother also experienced migraines for ten years and my younger sister, now forty, is experiencing the same symptom. I sought assistance from a Chinese herbalist for treatment and acupuncture. I haven't had a migraine since that treatment.

Because I was conscious of creating a harmonious workplace and environment, I don't recall mood changes to any great extent.

I turned sixty recently. It didn't worry me, although I don't bother to talk about my age. If people don't think I am sixty, well I am not going to tell them. I firmly believe what matters is your attitude, outlook on life and how you look after and present yourself, not age.

As I recall my adventures throughout my life I would probably describe myself as a 'late bloomer'. Opportunities emerged later in life, which I accepted, enjoyed and loved, and for me the good saying 'life begins at forty' really applied.

In the last five years I entered local government as a councillor and served two terms as mayor of our city. This did not make it any easier for me to control my weight, as I attended functions very frequently. I do admit that I do not do a great deal of exercise. Over the years I have participated in yoga, aerobics and tennis, but not on a regular basis.

Reflecting on how I felt, as I grew older and no longer able to have children, did not occupy a great deal of my time. I really enjoyed my babies and being a mother. Having babies was not easy for me. I experienced some life-threatening difficulties at childbirth, which caused us great worry and concern, and for that reason I would consider myself lucky to have had three healthy children. Even knowing the risks of childbirth, I resisted a hysterectomy for some years.

The reason for the hysterectomy was because I had experienced seven years of polycystic ovaries, severe pain and constant bleeding and discomfort. After the hysterectomy I felt very well, no discomfort at all, and regained my strength and energy. During this time I was prescribed the pill to relieve the symptoms, but I was unable to tolerate it.

I know some women I have met as a nurse feel that they have lost something when they have a hysterectomy. They feel they have lost an important part of themselves. Having the hysterectomy was regrettable to some extent, but, on the positive side, I felt so much better and free of pain it did not present to me as an issue.

Sexuality changes throughout life and is interesting to reflect upon. I have always felt feminine, and made a point of looking after myself. In comparing my sexuality before and after menopause, I would describe it as different, as was my state in life. In my thirties, with small children, I probably had more energy and more interest in sexuality. Now that I am postmenopausal, I don't feel the need to express sexuality in the same way. I experience a strong sense of closeness and completeness in my thirty-five-year marriage and relationship with my husband. I still have a great desire to be feminine and participate in life with energy and enthusiasm. You could say that 'the hormones may not be dancing' but other feelings and a sense of security provide me with energy and desire.

I have been fortunate to enjoy a successful career and happy family. We relax at Mount Martha where we have a holiday home and enjoy the company of our children, their friends and our family.

My husband has retired. He now looks after me. I think he has shouldered an enormous task! He now specialises in cooking. In his early cooking days I was presented with a different meal every night for six weeks. I looked forward to it each evening. He had never done this before and he has become quite skilled around the house. This is something I really enjoy and it allows me to enjoy my work. Our roles have reversed. There has been freedom in my life in the last few years. Our children are now independent and live away from home.

I have not placed a great deal of emphasis on managing my own finances. I probably haven't re-evaluated my financial state as much as I should have. I'm more aware of it now. It could be argued that I should have done it ten years ago, but for me it was not a priority. I am not driven to work for money, although the money did allow us to offer our children a good education. It does concern me when I hear staff say that they have to work and they do not enjoy it; in some cases they hate work. I often remind staff to do it because you want to, and put the money to good use. Enjoy it.

It is good to think about the next twenty years. Opportunities come our way that weren't available to our parents. It's altogether different. Lifestyles and expectations are different. Certainly, I would like to have grandchildren one day, when our children are ready. It will be another stage for us to enjoy. We would like to do some more travelling.

I intend to keep young even when I grow old. I am currently engaged in a wonderful challenge in establishing a new hospital with tertiary affiliation with Swinburne University. This hospital will be the first of its kind in Australia, where conventional orthodox medicine and scientifically validated natural therapies will be used. Some time in the future I may wish to contribute to some Boards. I have just finished five years participating in one of the Health Care Network Boards. That was an excellent experience. I enjoyed it. I have been Mayor of Boroondara Council. I have had two consecutive terms, of a year each, which is unusual. It is an honour and privilege to be in a position where I can help to effect change for the benefit of the community. I hope to stay in local council, as I do enjoy it. I think it is very stimulating, very challenging really. There is so much to be done in the community.

I think there are probably numerous things I have never thought about that I wouldn't mind having a go at.

I make a conscious effort to have a regular six monthly visit to my general practitioner and I make sure that I have a mammogram regularly, every two years. I do think women should take care of themselves. The interest and research in natural/complementary therapies is very popular, but I'm not taking anything of significance. Nutrition and healthy diet is important, and I am conscious of what I eat.

Overall, women have a great ability, they can do anything. They learn to master many skills. I'm not saying men can't, they just have a different way of doing things. In the workplace I have encouraged all staff to accept opportunities, maintain a balanced life with few regrets. This, I believe, is the way to a healthy mind and body.

Chapter Fifteen
Alzheimer's disease

The prevalence of Alzheimer's disease. Risk factors for developing Alzheimer's disease. Effects of oestrogen and hot flushes on the body in relation to the development of Alzheimer's. Studies into hormone replacement therapy and the prevention of Alzheimer's.

Alzheimer's disease is a common cause of dementia, accounting for about 72 per cent of cases of dementia. Other causes of dementia include cerebrovascular disease (16 per cent), Parkinson's disease (6 per cent), and miscellaneous causes (6 per cent).

The risk of developing Alzheimer's increases with age. A study of 32 000 people over the age of sixty-five in East Boston in the US found that 10.3 per cent of this population had probable Alzheimer's disease. In the age group sixty-five to seventy-four, the prevalence is 3 per cent, between seventy-five and eighty-four it is 18.7 per cent, and in those over eighty-five it is 47.7 per cent. Elderly women have a greater incidence of Alzheimer's disease than elderly men. Men may be protected from Alzheimer's disease through the conversion of testosterone to oestrogen in the brain.

Projecting from the East Boston study in 1980, it was estimated that there were 2.88 million people over the age of sixty-five with Alzheimer's disease in the US. By the year 2050, there will be 10.3 million people with

Alzheimer's disease. As a result, there will be a significant increase in the costs to the community in caring for them – mostly because many people with Alzheimer's disease are cared for in hostels or nursing homes. Of patients with Alzheimer's disease, 70 per cent die in nursing homes.

There appear to be multiple genetic, environmental and age-related factors that influence the onset of Alzheimer's disease. The process that leads to the end stage or final development of all the characteristics of Alzheimer's disease in elderly women may start after menopause, with the gradual development of pathological changes in the brain, in much the same way that fractures are the endstage event in osteoporosis. That is, the pre-clinical phase of Alzheimer's disease may be thirty years.

'It's extremely important, as an older woman, to have power and money, because if you don't have power and you don't have money you do get pushed into a corner.'

JEANNE PRATT

Risk factors for Alzheimer's disease include age, gender and a genetic disposition. An important source of oestrogen in the body in postmenopausal women comes by converting androstenodione, a hormone produced mainly in the adrenal gland, to oestrogen in adipose, or fatty, tissue. Obese women therefore tend to have higher oestrogen levels than thin women. Women with lower body weights tend to have a higher rate of Alzheimer's disease than obese women.

Alzheimer's disease is characterised by changes in cognitive function with loss of short-term memory, failure to grasp the meaning of complex situations and, later on, disorientation in time and space. The late stages of the disease include carelessness in dress, neglect of personal hygiene and incontinence.

Protective factors for Alzheimer's disease appear to include anti-inflammatory drugs, oestrogen and possibly antioxidants such as vitamin E and vitamin C.

Genetic factors may account for about 5 per cent of cases of Alzheimer's disease. The most intensive research has involved the apolipoprotein E gene. Individuals with this gene are more likely to have or develop the disease. Oestrogen has effects on a number of substances in the brain called neurotransmitters. These include acetylcholine, serotonin and norepinephrine. One of the features of Alzheimer's disease is loss of the neurotransmitter acetylcholine in regions of the brain that are involved in the learning and memory processes. This loss is related to the decrease in the levels of the enzyme acetylcholine transferase, which is involved in the production of acetylcholine. As well as its action on the neurotransmitters, oestrogen appears to play a role in the growth of nerve fibres in the brain.

Some scientists have investigated whether hot flushes may cause damage to a special area of the brain called the hippocampus. During the hot flush, there may be a decrease in blood flow to this area of the brain. The hippocampus is the area of the brain that is involved in verbal memory. This may explain why women who have taken hormone replacement therapy, even for a short period of time around the time of menopause for treatment of hot flushes, may have a lower rate of Alzheimer's disease later in life.

A relatively small number of clinical studies have evaluated the effects of oestrogen replacement therapy in the prevention and treatment of Alzheimer's disease. In assessing the outcomes of these studies, a number of possible confounding factors and biases should be considered. In general, oestrogen replacement therapy is used by women who are in the upper socio-economic groups, better educated, thinner and more physically active.

Nine case-control studies and two prospective cohort studies have evaluated the association between risk of Alzheimer's disease and postmenopausal oestrogen replacement therapy use.

A cohort is a group of people, some of whom have the risk factor or protective factor for the development of a disease and some who do not. They are usually observed over a long period of time – say twenty years – for the development of the disease that we are looking for. The case-control studies have produced conflicting results, with some studies showing a reduction in the risk of Alzheimer's disease with oestrogen replacement therapy use.

Case-control studies look at people who have the disease now and look backwards to see if they have taken the risk factor for the disease or not. Others indicate an increased risk or a non-significant effect.

The conflicting results may be the result of differences in the collection of information about oestrogen use, recall bias and possible misclassification of cases. It is important when doctors are diagnosing Alzheimer's disease that they compare symptoms with the proper diagnostic guidelines.

'The menopause is something all women experience and unless we can talk about it openly we will never be able to get women to realise it's not something we need to suffer in silence. It's a fact of life and a very important one.'

ITA BUTTROSE

Recently an important study was published in the *Journal of the American Medical Association*. This study was conducted on 120 postmenopausal women with mild to moderate Alzheimer's disease. It was a one-year randomised, placebo-controlled, double-blinded trial in which patients were required to have had a hysterectomy, because the trial used treatment with oestrogen alone for one year. Progestins added to oestrogen replacement therapy may have negated the effect on cognition in women using oestrogen replacement therapy.

The participants were randomly assigned to taking either oestrogen, 0.625 mg/d (n=42), 2.25 mg/d (n=39), or a similar appearing placebo (an inactive, but similar appearing medication (n=39). Follow-up was at two, six, twelve and fifteen months.

Overall, oestrogen failed to improve cognition or functional outcomes in women with mild to moderate Alzheimer's disease and hysterectomies.

This study is superior to the clinical trials mentioned earlier using oestrogen replacement therapy for Alzheimer's disease. The number of women involved in the study, the length of the study, the use of two dose levels, and the multicentre recruitment enhances the likelihood that the results indicate that oestrogen replacement therapy may not be useful in the treatment of women who already have Alzheimer's disease.

In other words, once the damage has occurred in the brain, it may not be possible to reverse it. This is why there are many studies being conducted around the world that are looking at a wide range of medications, including oestrogen, which may prevent the damage starting or continuing in the brains of susceptible people.

Larger randomised, controlled, long-term studies are needed to evaluate the effects of oestrogen in Alzheimer's disease. The Women's Health Initiative trial has recently included a dementia component. It has sufficient numbers of women in the study to answer many questions about oestrogen replacement therapy in the prevention of Alzheimer's disease.

It is hoped it will determine the role of oestrogen replacement therapy in the prevention of Alzheimer's disease. In this study, approximately 8,000 women will be treated for ten years. The outcome will be available in the year 2007.

Appendix
The interview questions

The purpose of this interview is to ascertain through a series of questions the changes women have gone through in the perimenopausal and postmenopausal years, i.e. late forties to late fifties. We note that with this publication we try to convey and portray a positive image of women for this age group, and how they have coped with their successful careers and family life despite the physiological and psychological changes that occur.

1   Tell me about the years leading to menopause.

2   What were your feelings and thoughts going through menopause? Were there certain factors that concerned you (e.g. lack of energy, unreproductive years, loss of libido)?

3   Did you discuss any of the changes you were experiencing with your family and friends?

4   Did they provide you with any support?

5   How did you cope with your business or at work.

6   Did it have a dramatic effect on what you did?

7   Did going through menopause affect any of your daily activities?

8   Were you concerned about growing old?

9   Did you notice any physical changes and loss of energy and were they disturbing to you? (e.g. weight gain) Did you suffer any mood changes and, if so, how did they affect you?

10   Tell me about the positive aspects of going through menopause (e.g. no more birth control, no more periods, control of sexuality).

11   How is your general health and wellbeing now compared to the years leading to menopause?

12   Was menopause a time when you felt a need to re-evaluate
     – lifestyle issues
     – relationships with family and friends
     – financial states
     – career

13   What are you hoping to achieve in the next twenty to thirty years?

14   Is this period of your life different to any other stage of life (compared to before menopause and to when you felt much younger)?

15   Do you follow any special diet or exercise program?

16   Do you have regular medical check-ups such as pap smears and mammograms?

17   Is HRT (or other alternative medications) something that you have taken or would consider taking?

References

1997. Food, Nutrition and the Prevention of Cancer: a Global Perspective. World Cancer Research Fund in association with American Institute for Cancer Research. Washington, DC: 254, 270.

1998. Life after HERS: a Menopause Management Q&A Report. *Menopause Management* 7 (6): 7–12.

Albertazzi, P. *et al.* 1998. The effect of dietary soy supplementation on hot flushes. *Obstetrics and Gynecology* 91 (1): 6–11.

Alberts, D. S. *et al.* 2000. Lack of effect of a high-fiber cereal supplement on the recurrence of colorectal adenomas. *New England Journal of Medicine.* 342 (16): 1156–62.

Anderson, J. *et al.* 1995. Meta-analysis of the effects of soy protein intake on serum lipids. *New England Journal of Medicine* 335 (5): 276–82.

Andersson, B. *et al.*1997. Estrogen replacement therapy decreases hyperandrogenicity and improves glucose homeostasis and plasma lipids in postmenopausal women with non-insulin-dependent diabetes melitus. *Journal of Clinical Endocrinology and Metabolism* 82: 638–43.

Asthana, S. *et al.* 1999. Cognitive and neuroendocrine response to transdermal estrogen in postmenopausal women with Alzheimer's disease: results of a placebo-controlled, double blind, pilot study. *Psychoneuroendocrinology* 24 (6): 657–77.

Australian Diabetes, Obesity and Lifestyle Study (AusDiab) 2000. International Diabetes Institute.

Barnes, S. 1998, Phytoestrogens and breast cancer. *Baillieres Clinical Endocrinology & Metabolism* 12 (4), 559–79.

Barraclough, B. H. 1994. Breast lumps: some questions answered. *Modern Medicine of Australia*.18–28.

Barrett-Connor, E. and T. L. Bush. 1991. Estrogen and coronary heart disease in women. *Journal of the American Medical Association* 265 (14): 1861–7.

Berger, G. 1999. Abstract. Menopause and culture: a cross-cultural analysis of Australian and Filipino women's experience. 3rd Australian Menopause Society Conference.

Birge, S. 1997. The role of ovarian hormones in cognition and dementia. *Neurology* 48 (suppl. l7): S1: 81–7.

Birge, S. J. 1996. Is there a role for estrogen replacement therapy in the prevention and treatment of dementia. *Journal of the American Gerontology Association* 44: 865–70.

Black, D. M. *et al*. 1996. Randomised trial of effect of alendronate on risk of fracture in women with existing vertebral fractures. *Lancet* 348: 1535–41.

Boulet, M. J. *et al*. 1994. Climacteric and menopause in seven south-east Asian countries. *Maturitas* 16: 157–76.

Brandi, M. L. 1997. Natural and synthetic isoflavones in the prevention and treatment of chronic diseases. *Calcified Tissue International* 61 (suppl. 11): S5–8.

Breast Cancer in Australian Women 1921–1994. NHMRC National Breast Cancer Centre, Australian Institute Of Health and Welfare:13.

Brenner, D. E. *et al*. 1994. Postmenopausal replacement therapy and the risk of Alzheimer's Disease: A population-based case control study. *American Journal of Epidemiology* 149 (3): 262–7.

Broe, G. A. *et al*. 1990. A case-control study of Alzheimer's disease in Australia. *Neurology* 40: 1698–707.

Brussaard, H. E. *et al*. 1997. Effect of 17 beta-estradiol on plasma lipids and LDL oxidation in postmenopausal women with type 2 diabetes mellitus. *Artherioscleosis, Thrombosis and Vascular Biology* 17: 324–30.

Bush, T. L. *et al*. 1996. Effects of hormone therapy on bone mineral density: results from the Postmenopausal Estrogen/Progestin Interventions (PEPI) trial. *Journal of the American Medical Association* 276 (17): 1389–96.

Buzdar, A. U. and G. N. Hortobagyi. 1999. Recent advances in adjuvant therapy of breast cancer. *Seminars in Oncology* 26 (4 suppl. 12): 21–7.

Cameron, J. D. and A. M. Dart. 1994. Exercise training increases total systemic arterial compliance in humans. *American Journal of Physiology* 266 (2Pt2): H693–701.

Chen, R. Q. *et al*. 1999. The role of specific Chinese herbal medicine in the management of vasomotor symptoms in Australian postmenopausal women. *Third Australian Menopause Society Congress*, Cairns.

Cohen, S. *et al.* 1999. Risedronate therapy prevents corticosteroid- induced bone loss. *Arthritis and Rheumatism* 42 (11): 2309–18.

Colditz, G. A. *et al.* 1995. The use of estrogens and progestins and the risk of breast cancer in postmenopausal women. *New England Journal of Medicine* 332 (21): 1489–593.

Collaborative Group on Hormonal Factors in Breast Cancer. 1997. Breast cancer and hormone replacement therapy: collaborative reanalysis of data from 51 epidemiological studies of 52,705 women with breast cancer and 108,411 without breast cancer. *Lancet* 450: 1047–59.

Cummings, S. R. *et al.* 1997. Effect of alendronate on risk of fracture in women with low bone density but without vertebral fractures: results from the Fracture Intervention Trial. *Archives of Internal Medicine* 157: 2617–24.

Cummings, S. R. *et al.* 1999. The effect of raloxifene on risk of breast cancer in postmenopausal women. *Journal of the American Medical Association* 1281 (23): 2189–97.

De jong, P. C. and G. H. Blijham. 1999. New aromatase inhibitors for the treatment of advanced breast cancer in postmenopausal women. *Netherlands Journal of Medicine* 55 (2): 50–8.

Dennerstein, L. *et al.* 1993. Menopausal symptoms in Australian women. *Medical Journal of Australia* 159 (4): 232–6.

Ettinger, B. *et al.* 1999. Reduction of vertebral fracture risk in postmenopausal women with osteoporosis treated with raloxifene. *Journal of the American Medical Association* 282: 637–45.

Feingold, K. R. and M. D. Siperstein. 1986. Diabetes vascular disease. *Advances in Internal Medicine* 31: 309–40.

Fillit, H. *et al.* 1986. Observations in a preliminary open trial of Estradiol Therapy for Senile Dementia-Alzheimer's type. *Psychoneuroendocrinology* 11 (3): 337–45.

Fisher, B. 1999. Highlights of the recent National Surgical Adjuvant Breast and Bowel Project studies in the treatment and prevention of breast cancer. *Ca: a Cancer Journal for Clinicians* 49 (3): 159–77.

Friday, K. E. 1998. Estrogen replacement therapy improves glycemic control and high density lipoprotein cholesterol concentrations in postmenopausal type 2 diabetic women. Abstract. *Diabetes* 47 (suppl. 1): A357.

Graves, A. R. *et al.* 1990. A case-control study of Alzheimer's disease. *Annals of Neurology* 28: 766–74.

Grodstein, F. *et al.* 1996. Postmenopausal estrogen and progestin use and the risk of cardiovascular disease. *New England Journal of Medicine* 335 (7): 453–61.

Grodstein, F. *et al.* 1996. Prospective study of exogenous hormones and risk of pulmonary embolism in women. *Lancet* 348: 983–7.

Grodstein, F. *et al.* 1997. Postmenopausal hormone therapy and mortality. *New England Journal of Medicine* 336 (25): 1769–75.

Grodstein, F. *et al.* 1998. Postmenopausal hormone use and risk for colorectal cancer and adenoma. *Annals of Internal Medicine* 128 (9): 705–12.

Harris, S. T. *et al.* 1999. Effects of Risedronate treatment on vertebral and nonvertebral fractures in women with postmenopausal osteoporosis. A randomized clinical trial. *Journal of the American Medical Association* 282 (14): 1344–52.

Heikkinen, J. *et al.*1991. Moderate exercise does not enhance the positive effect of estrogen on bone mineral density in postmenopausal women. *Calcified Tissue International* 49 (suppl.): S83–4.

Henderson, V. W. 1994. Estrogen replacement therapy in older women: comparisons between Alzheimer's disease and nondemented control subjects. *Archives Neurology* 51: 896–900.

Henderson, V. W. *et al.* 2000. Estrogen for Alzheimer's disease in women: randomized, double-blind, placebo-controlled trial. *Neurology* 54 (2): 295–301.

Heyman, A. *et al.* 1984. Alzheimer's disease: a study of epidemiological aspects. *Annals of Neurology* 15: 335–41.

Hirata, J. D. *et al.* 1997. Does dong quai have estrogenic effects in postmenopausal women? A double blind, placebo-controlled trial. *Fertility and Sterility* 68: 981–6.

Hochberg, M. 2000. Preventing fractures in postmenopausal women with osteoporosis. *Drugs and Aging* (4) 317–30.

Hodgson, J. M. *et al.* 1998. Supplementation with bioflavonoid phytoestrogens does not alter serum lipid concentration – a randomised controlled trial in humans. *Journal of Nutrition* 128 (4): 728–32.

Honisett, S. *et al.* 2001. The effect of exercise and hormone replacement therapy on bone parameters (manuscript in preparation)

Honjo, H. *et al.* 1989. In vivo effects by estrone sulphate on the central nervous system-senile dementia (Alzheimer's type) j. steroid *Biochemistry* 34: 521–5.

Honjo, H. *et al.* 1993. An effect of conjugated estrogen to cognitive impairment in women with senile-dementia Alzheimer's type: a placebo-controlled double blind study. *Journal of the Japanese Menopause Society* 1: 167–71.

Howes, L. 1999. Isoflavone, phyto-estrogens. *Medical Observer* (March).

Hulley, S. *et al.* 1998. Randomized trial of estrogen plus progestins for secondary prevention of coronary heart disease in postmenopausal women. *Journal of the American Medical Association* 280 (7) : 605–13.

Ingram, D. *et al.* 1997. Case-control study of phytoestrogens and breast cancer. *Lancet* 350: 990–4.

Isles, C. G. *et al.* 1992. Relation between coronary risk and coronary mortality in women of the Refrew and Paisley survey: comparison with men. *Lancet* 339: 702–5.

Ismael, N. N. 1994. A study on the menopause in Malaysia. *Maturatas* 19: 205–9.

Jones, G. *et al.* 1994. Symptomatic fracture incidence in elderly men and women: the Dubbo Osteoporosis Epidemiology Study (DOES). *Osteoporosis International* 4 (5): 227–82.

Kashiwa, A. and J. Rippe. 1987. *Fitness walking for women.* Berkley Publishing Group.

Kawas, C. *et al.* A prospective study of estrogen replacement therapy and the risk of developing Alzheimer's Disease: the Baltimore Study of Aging. *Neurology* 197 (48): 1517–21.

Knight, D. C. and J. A. Eden. 1995. Phytoestrogens – a short review. *Maturitus* 22: 167–75.

Kohrt, W. M. *et al.*1997. Effects of exercise involving predominantly either joint-reaction or ground reaction forces on bone mineral density in older women. *Journal of Bone Mineral Research* 12 (8): 1253–61.

Kuller, L. H. 1996. Hormone replacement therapy and its potential relationship to dementia. *Journal of the American Gerontology Society* 44 (7): 878–80.

Lindheim, S.R. *et al.* 1994. The independent effects of exercise and estrogen on lipids and lipoproteins in postmenopausal women. *Obstetrics and Gynecology* 83 (2): 167–72.

Lock, M. 1994. Menopause in cultural context. *Experimental Gerontology* 29: 307–17.

Love, S. 1997. *Hormone Book.* Random House.

Lufkin, E. G. 1992. Treatment of postmenopausal osteoporosis with transdermal estrogen. *Annals of Internal Medicine* 117: 1–9.

MacLennan, A. H. *et al.* 1999. Hormone replacement therapies in women at risk of cardiovascular disease and osteoporosis in South Australia in 1997. *Medical Journal of Australia* 170 (11): 524–7.

Manson, J. E. *et al.* 1992. A prospective study of postmenopasal estrogen therapy and subsequent incidence of non-insulin dependent diabetes mellitus. *Annals of Epidemiology* 2: 665–73.

McCarthy, T. 1994. The prevalence of symptoms in menopausal women in the far East: Singapore segment. *Maturatas* 19: 199–204.

McClung, M. R. *et al.* 2001. Effect of risedronate on the risk of hip fracture in elderly women. *New England Journal of Medicine* 344 (5): 333–40.

McPherson, K. *et al.* 1995. Breast Cancer – Epidemiology, Risk Factors, and Genetics. *ABC of Breast Diseases.* Ed. J. M. Dixon. BMJ Publishing Group: 18–21.

Meade, T. W. 1999. HERS and its aftermath. Editorial. *Menopause Management* 7 (6): 2–5.

Messina, M. 1999. Soyfoods, soybeans, phytoestrogens (isoflavones) and bone health. *9th International Menopause Society World Congress on the Menopause Proceedings,* Japan.

Meunier, P. J. 1999. Evidence-based medicine and osteoporosis: A comparison of fracture risk reduction data from osteoporosis randomised clinical trials. *International Journal of Clinical Practice* 53 (2): 122–9.

Miller, J. B. 2000. *The GI Factor.* Hodder.

Morris, M. C. *et al.* 1998. Vitamin E and vitamin C supplement use and risk of incident Alzheimer's disease. *Alzheimer's Disease and Associated disorders* 12 (3): 121–6.

Mortel, K. F. and J. S. Meyer. 1995. Lack of postmenopausal replacement therapy and the risk of dementia. *Journal of Neuropsychiatry Clinical Neuroscience* 7: 334–7.

Mulnard, R. A. 2000. Estrogen Replacement Therapy for Treatment of Mild to Moderate Alzheimer Disease. A Randomized Controlled Trial. *Journal of the American Medical Association* 283 (8): 1007–15.

Murkies, A. L. *et al.* 1995. Dietary flour supplementation decreases postmenopausal hot flushes: effect of soy and wheat. *Maturitas* 21: 189–95.

Murkies, A. L. *et al.* 1998. Clinical review 92–Phytoestrogens. *Journal of Clinical Endocrinology and Metabolism* 83 (2): 297–303.

Nelson, M. E. 1997. *Strong Women Stay Young.* Lothian / Aurum Press.

Nelson, M. E. and S. Warnick. 2000. *Strong Women, Strong Bones.* Lothian.

Nelson, M. E. *et al.* 1994. Effects of high-intensity strength training on multiple risk factors for osteoporotic fractures. *Journal of the American Medical Association* 272 (24): 1909–14.

Nestel, P. *et al.* 1997. Soy isoflavones improve systemic arterial compliance but not plasma lipids in menopausal and perimenopausal women. *Arteriosclerosis, Thrombosis and Vascular Biology* 17: 3392–8.

Nevitt, M. C. *et al.* 2000. Effect of alendronate on limited-activity days and bed-disability days caused by back pain in postmenopausal women with existing vertebral fractures. *Archives Internal Medecine* 160: 77–85

Oddens, B. J. and M. J. Boulet. 1997. Hormone replacement therapy among Danish women aged 45–65 years – prevalence, determinants and compliance. *Obstetrics and Gynecology* 90 (2): 269–77.

Onkura, T. *et al.* 1994. Evaluation of estrogen treatment in female patients with dementia of the Alzheimer's type. *Endocrinology J* 41: 361–71.

Onkura, T. O. *et al.* 1994. Low-dose estrogen replacement therapy for Alzheimer's Disease in women. Menopause. *Journal of the North American Medical Society* 1 (3): 125–30.

Osuntokun, Bo *et al.* 1992. Alzheimer's disease in Nigeria. *African Journal of Medicine and Medical Sciences* 21 (2): 71–7.

Paganini-Hill, A. and V. W. Henderson. 1994. Estrogen deficiency and risk of Alzheimer's disease in women. *American Journal of Epidemiology* 140 (3): 256–61.

Pinder, S. E. *et al.* 1999. Ductal carcinoma in situ of the human breast. *Annali Italiani di Chirurgia* 70 (3): 434–7.

Prince, R.L. *et al.* 1991. Prevention of postmenopausal osteoporosis. A comparative study of exercise, calcium supplementation and hormone replacement therapy. *New England Journal of Medicine* 325 (17): 1189–95.

Reginster, J. Y. *et al.* 2000. Randomised trial of the effects of risedronate on vertebral fractures in women with established postmenopausal osteoporosis. *Osteoporosis International* 11: 83–91.

Richards, M. A. *et al.* 1999. Influence of delay on the survival in patients with breast cancer: a systematic review. *Lancet* 353 (9159): 1119–26.

Rose, D. P. *et al.* 1986. International comparisons of mortality rates for cancer of the breast, ovary, prostate and colon, and per capita food consumption. *Cancer* 58 (11): 2363–71.

Ryan, H. 1999. *Menopause across culture.* Mid-Link Menopause Service.

Samil, S. R. and S.W. Wishuwardhani. 1994. Health of Indonesian women city-dwellers of perimenopausal age. *Maturatas* 19: 191–7.

Sang, K. G. *et al.* 1998. Alendronate for the prevention and treatment of glucosteroid-induced osteoporosis. Glucosteroid-induced osteoporosis intervention study group. *New England Journal of Medicine* 339: 292–9.

Schatzkin, A. *et al.* 2000. Lack of effect of a low-fat, high-fiber diet on the recurrence of colorectal adenomas. *New England Journal of Medicine* 342 (16): 1149–55.

Schnitzer, T. *et al.* 2000. Therapeutic equivalence of alendronate 70mg once-weekly and alendronate 10mg daily in the treatment of osteoporosis. *Aging Clinical Experimental Research* 12 (1): 1–12.

Sharma, V. K. and M. L. S. Saxena. 1981. Climacteric symptoms: a study in the Indian context. *Maturatas* 3: 11–20.

Sharp, R. 1999. Natural HRT: are women getting what they think? *Medical Observer* (February).

Smith, E. L. and C. Gilligan. 1991. Physical activity effects on bone metabolism. *Calcified Tissue International* 49: S50–4.

Stampfer, M. J. and G. A. Colditz. 1991. Estrogen replacement therapy and coronary heart disease: a quantitative assessment of the epidemiological evidence. *Preventative Medicine* 20: 47–63.

Stoppard, M. 1994. *Menopause*. Viking.

Strauss, L. *et al.* 1998. Dietary phytoestrogens and their role in the hormonally dependent disease. *Toxicology Letters* 102–3: 349–54.

Tang, M. X. *et al.* 1996. Effect of postmenopausal estrogen during menopause on risk and age at onset of Alzheimer's disease. *Lancet* 348: 429–32.

Tuck, C. H. 1999. Benefits and risks of HRT for menopausal women with diabetes. *North American Menopause Society, Proceedings*.

Ueda, K. *et al.* 1992. Prevalence and etiology of dementia in a Japanese community. *Stroke* 23 (6): 798–803.

Waddell, T. K. *et al.* 1999. Withdrawal of hormonal therapy for 4 weeks decreases arterial compliance in postmenopausal women. *Journal of Hypertension* 17 (3): 413–18.

Waring, S. C. *et al.* 1999. Postmenopausal estrogen replacement therapy and the risk of AD: a population-based study. *Neurology* 52 (5): 965–70.

Whitehouse, P. J. 1997. Genesis of Alzheimer's disease The role of ovarian hormones in cognition and dementia. *Neurology* 48 (suppl. 17): S1: 81–7.

World Health Organisation, 1993. *World Health Statistics 1992*, Geneva.

Writing group for the PEPI trial. 1995. Effects of estrogen or estrogen/progestin regimens on heart disease risk factors in postmenopausal women. *Journal of the American Medical Association* 273 (3): 199–208.

Yaffe, K. *et al.* 1998. Estrogen therapy in postmenopausal women – effects on cognitive function and dementia. *Journal of the American Medical Association* 279 (9).

Index